Dear Readers,

It is no easy task to publish a written a
it was easier for me to write this book.
of publishing was beyond my paper money budget and could not be paid for in the currency in which I am truly rich: love and joy.

I therefore listened to my soul and decided to step onto the path least travelled and try and do it all myself. To see what I was truly capable of with this book. A book handed to me by the creative universe that exists within me.

The stories told by nature are true stories. Told by them to me throughout my lifetime. The Yoga knowledge is a culmination of living and studying as a Yogi for 17 years. The editing, design, interior set up, and audio recordings have all been done to the best of my ability. Only the proofreading was done by an amazing soul by the name of Heather. Her editing of this book, from a foundation of love for it, helped create the magic you are about to read. She is truly an amazing soul.

Therefore, please excuse any errors into which you may bump. Try to forgive them and see past the surface into the magic of the content.

A little like life, where we keep focusing on the superficial, while sacrificing what is important: what is inside.

Thank you for trusting me with your body, mind, and soul and for the journey on which we are about to embark. The journey into the magic and power that lives in you.

Namaste. Sheena

(https://heathersteinphd.com)

This book is dedicated to

Corey whose love for me & desire for change inspired this book

Paola & Sonia who loved & talked me through this whole book

My mother (Bhagavti Patel) who literally saved my life with her love and allowed me to be me

Raiden, Rayah & Aadi, my rays of light, and every other child in the world who deserve us to be better humans

Every one of my teachers over the last seventeen years, who kept moving me forward on this journey

ALL my students for whom I took this journey, so you too could find the courage to change

Everyone who has taken the time to write down the knowledge of Yoga

&

Every human who seeks to know their true selves

Table of Contents

HUMAN COLLIDES WITH THE UNIVERSE	3
HUMAN MEETS YOGA	12
NATURE WELCOMES THE HUMAN	22
OCEAN EXPLAINS CONSCIOUSNESS	34
THE ELEPHANT & THE HUMAN MIND	52
HUMAN SUFFERING & THE STARS	67
THE EAGLE & THE HUMAN PERSONALITY	85
DESTINY & THE JOURNEY INTO CHANGE	99
YAMAS & THE LEOPARD	112
THE ENORMOUS RESTRAINTS	121
BUTTERFLY OBSERVES THE HUMAN	130
MASCULINE & FEMININE: BIGGER THAN A PENIS OR VAGINA	142
YOGA ASANAS: GETTING HIGH OFF YOUR OWN BODY	157
ASANAS PRACTISED BY ORANGUTAN	168
THE MAGIC OF DOING NOTHING: A LION'S WORLD	181
PRANA, THE FORGOTTEN ONE	192
HOW BREATH WORKS: THE TREES SPEAK	204
TAMING THE DRUNKEN MONKEY MIND	214
GOODBYE ILLUSION, HELLO UNIVERSE	225
THE AWAKENING	233

1

Human Collides with the Universe

In every tragedy and trauma there is a gift of knowledge and light just as in every gain, there is a loss that furthers that knowledge.

"I met a human today."

"You met a what?" squawked my friend Hawk, who sat perched beside me.

"I believe she said a human," laughed the three-thousand-year-old Baobab tree on which the three of us sat. The third being Leopard, who lay splayed across Baobab's thick branches.

"What do you mean 'met'? And why do you look like you have gulped too much oxygen?" queried the turquoise Ocean, its waves lapping below us.

"Well, I was flying along Ocean, trying to catch the one fish that meets my daily survival need, when suddenly, our buddy Wind changed its direction and blew me over a cliff and into a human. He was sitting under a tree with his legs crossed and seemed to be engaged in the human act of prayer. What a magnificent specimen of human he was: blue-eyed, broad-chested, two arms, two legs, and a smile that made my wings wilt. Their bodies are a splendid creation in the multitude of ways they can experience this Earth. But so is their ignorance of how they can experience this Universe for a limited time in a form that is so unique."

"Oh bother," smiled Hawk. "You do know that this is never going to work? Humans, don't even think they are a species, let alone part of nature."

"You got that right," muttered Baobab. "I always hear them talking underneath me about this species and that species as if we exist on a different plane almost as if they themselves are not a species. But that is not the worst of it. They keep blabbing on about nature, unaware that they are a part of the very definition of nature.

Eagle, ask your blue-eyed human, the next time you are having an interspecies chat, who exactly do they think they are? If they do not see themselves as connected to us, then what are they?"

"You plan to meet him again?" stretched Leopard, almost causing him to roll right off Baobab and into Ocean.

"I have no choice. Universe spoke to me in the silence between my breaths and told me the time has come to explain Yoga and the Universe to the Human. It is the only way to ensure the survival of all of us for we have entered *Kali Yuga*, the age of darkness, vice, and misery. If humans do not connect to their true selves and, by extension, to us, life as we know it will end. Plus, I think I may have a little crush on this human; their form is so interesting." I mumbled into the wind. My fellow energetic forms would think I had completely lost my animal brain.

"Eagle, snap out of it. You know we can hear your mind. And honestly, you are not saying what we all want to know," flowed Ocean. "What did the two of you speak about?"

"Many things." I hopped about, "but mostly I tried to explain to him that he and I were the same, united in our consciousness and born from the same intelligent universe that pervades all of us. I shared with him that all living beings are merely vibrating intelligent energies, each with their own essence and history that started long before they entered their present-day form. What separated us was our forms, the human one being the most complex of all of nature's forms.

Which they think makes them smart, but I know it just layers them with ignorance. It keeps moving them further away from their soul or 'pure consciousness,' as some of them like to call it."

At this, we all burst out into such a tidal wave of laughter that the mycelium below Earth and all the animals housed in

Ocean's large and fabulous body felt the vibration. And soon all of nature was laughing with us, except humans because their egos and conditioned mind had buried their connection to the rest of us.

"What exactly did you tell him?" asked Butterfly, who had brought all its majestic colours and elegance to this confluence of energies.

"Well, once he got over the shock that he and I could converse and he looked beyond my sexy feathered body, it went something like this:

'Now Corey, I am going to tell you a story. If you allow yourself to listen to the whole story with an open mind and heart, it will change your life forever. In the beginning, it will seem gigantic and implausible. However, by the end of it, what seemed impossible will transform into the possible. It is not a story based on any religion, caste, colour, nationality, or any of the other major categories by which you humans define yourselves. No, it is a story that will take you on a journey into yourself. A journey that will reconnect you to your true conscious self, so you may learn to live a life of peace and joy. No, it is not a fairy tale, a myth, or a fantasy. It is, in fact, the true story of Yoga.

But first, let's start with the foundations of this story. Imagine a blank screen as big as the world. Now imagine that screen is filled with trillions and trillions of vibrating dots, each representing intelligent conscious energy. You know, just how the television set looked back in the day when all the programming was done and the screen turned into thousands of vibrating dots."

I paused for a moment feeling the warmth and love of the deep orange glamourous Sun beginning to rise, adding light to the place at which we all met.

"Well go on," nudged Hawk, stretching its majestic wings.

"Okay, so are you imagining the screen with all the vibrating dots." They all nodded in unison, although Leopard's head was so big it nearly fell off Baobab again when the tree nodded its branches as well.

"Now take a stick and start to draw shapes on it, the shape of trees, birds, animals, oceans, clouds, and, yes, even the human."

As he visualised that, I explained to him that everything in the Universe, of which Earth is a part, is just vibrating energy at different frequencies in different forms. All of us are part of the same screen. It is just our form and essence that is different. Erase the form, and we are back to vibrating across the screen seeking a new form."

"So, let me get this right," sang Butterfly. "All we are is energy, and this fabulous body I live in is just a house for my energy. Remove my house, and my consciousness, which is energy, lives on. So, really, it is only our forms and the frequency at which we are vibrating that differentiate us. Energetically we are all connected, and therefore the actions of each of us, affect all of us."

"Yes siree," I fluttered. "All of us are just energy, and in that energy, our consciousness is held. When we plug into it, we can talk to everyone, dolphins, flowers, Earth, the entire Universe, just as we are doing in this moment because each of us are part of the same screen. We were all birthed by the Universe. Therefore, the DNA of the Universe is in all of us, and all we, well, they the human, must do is access it."

"Woah. Back up there, miss Eagle," swayed Baobab. "You had me until you got to that Universe stuff. Please explain that to me. The other day I had these humans leaning against my trunk AUMing and thanking the Universe as if it existed in our friend Sky and was therefore separate from them. They treated it as if it were an object."

Human Collides with the Universe

I started to hop along the branch all excited, so excited that I hopped right off the branch. I flew over Ocean, dived in, felt Ocean's energy dance with mine, and then rocketed back up to the branch.

"You may all want to do a salutation and move your energy because this is big, and your tiny happy animal brains may just explode," I laughed at my friends. And so, they all moved in their own unique way, each salutation influenced by the limitations of the body that housed them. When they were done, they all settled back down to a listening position.

Ahh, the Human. For a moment I allowed myself to settle on his shoulder and feel his energy, as I had that very morning, not far from the place I was born, a nest filled with all the trash that humans threw onto Earth as if Earth did not have feelings or value. Yet they had taken Earth to be theirs and theirs alone and split it, created boundaries, and then sold it or distributed it! Then they told other humans what boundaries they could and could not cross. Can you imagine if all the species on the planet did that? For sure Earth would kick our fabulous natural bottoms for being so presumptuous as to behave as if she belonged to anyone.

"You are right about that," bellowed Earth from below. "Eagle, you keep forgetting we can all read your mind. Please keep your feathers on when dreaming about the Human. But you are right. I am tired of humans and their conditioned belief that I belong to them and them alone and that they can cut my trees, kill my animals, dam and pollute all my water bodies, attempt to sell my ground, and basically treat me as if they gave rise to me and not the other way around. As if I were manifested just to pander to their needs and no one else's! They forget that I birthed them as well."

"Amen to that," Ocean splashed. "Of all the Universe's manifestations, I am slightly bamboozled by the human. However, I feel that by the end of this story Eagle shall give us all a little more insight into the human. After all, Yoga did arrive to bring the human back into the fold of nature by reconnecting them with the Universe that resides within. So, tell us, Eagle, how exactly did you explain to handsome human the Universe?"

"Well, as we perched on the cliff overlooking Ocean, with only a breath between us, I told him this....

'Once upon a time, the consciousness of the Universe, which we shall call The Universe, or the masculine Purusha, collided with nature, the feminine Prakriti. Prior to this entanglement, nature, defined as force upon matter, lay in a slumber; it was completely balanced. Each of its three *gunas* lay still as there was no force being presented on any of them. When the Universe collided into force it awoke each of the *gunas*, which created a vibration in matter. That vibration was AUM.

In that vibration, the *gunas* ignited themselves into movement and gave rise to the five elements and all of creation. There was the *rajasic guna*, which sought to create and move, the *sattvic guna*, which sought balance and peace, and the *tamasic guna*, which by its very nature gave rise to death and transformation. Each was a force of their own that constantly intertwined with the other to give rise to all of creation and the cycle of life and death.

As Earth formed, it also gave rise to multitudes of living beings, including humans, which we shall henceforth call 'nature.' Each is made up of varying portions of the five elements and all the *gunas*. As a result, all of nature is constantly shifting, changing, transforming, and evolving as each *guna* seeks to find balance with the other two. Hence why volcanoes erupt, hurricanes occur, living beings continually shift and change, and so forth; they are all seeking to come back into balance.

Now, intertwined in all this nature was the Universe that had become entangled in it upon collision. The result of this entanglement was that consciousness had entered every living being to experience that which it had assisted in creating.

Human Collides with the Universe

The Universe is a genius, made up of intelligence, love, and the radiance of light that manifested itself as conscious energy. Its intelligence is seen in every living being's ability to adapt, flow, and survive in the constant impermanence of nature. In every being except the human, consciousness manifested itself clearly as the ability of living beings to connect with all of nature's energy force, to hear it, read it, and survive within it without attaching to the impermanence of it, but rather flowing with it and accepting death and live life according to their purpose.

However, in the human the magnitude and complexity of nature was so large that consciousness was buried, so it remained invisible to most them. Yet, of all the planet's creations, it was the human form that had evolved as the most sophisticated being and became the only form conscious of itself with a sense of I AM. At least that we know of.

As a result, it was only in the human being that the individual soul was able to purify itself of karmas and impressions that had been grooved into it from past and present actions and be aware of itself. However, for the soul, the observer of all, to be able to see itself in the reflection of a clean and pure human mind, it had to clean the mind of all impurities. As only then was the soul able to guide the human form; to create, to move forward with its own evolution and that of the universe. As well as to experience all of nature's magnificence without being entangled in it.

At this, Corey burst out into laughter and looked at me. 'So, let me guess: you are now going to tell me that you, the stunning Eagle, are smarter than me, the Human, part of the species that has invented the rocket, the spaceship, Internet, and vaccines because you lead with your soul and we with our mind.'

Being a bird and all, I was unfamiliar with human sarcasm and amazed at how smart he was being for a human. He already acknowledged my Purusha was smarter than all his Prakritis, his senses, mind, etc. So, I replied, 'Yes, of course I am, and you are a genius for recognizing that, but it is not as simple as that.'

Yoga, Where the Impossible Meets the Possible

I am not sure why he looked so bamboozled, but I guessed it was because the concept of the Universe was just too big for him. So I continued trying to explain it to him.

'The Universe, or infinite space, is filled with frequencies that carry information. It is a mind but not the shallow frivolous mind with which you humans identify. Instead, the word most often used to describe the MIND and LIFE that is the Universe is 'God'.

The Universe is a single field of information where there is no time, where polarities and dualities become one, where there is no separation or division, where everything you ever need to know exists. It is where your pure consciousness lives on long after your body, your form has died.

Do you know there were these human scientists who did this experiment where they increased the vibration of two photons in a vacuum? They believed that if they were truly separate from each other, then when one photon disappeared, the other would disappear soon after it. But what happened surprised the pants off them, metaphorically speaking of course. They both disappeared at the exact same time because there is no separation between anything.

I can tell from the look on your face that you are a little lost, and of course you are, this topic is huge. It is why I need to explain all the pieces for you to fully understand the whole.'

'So, I will meet you again?' he asked, piercing my soul with his blue eyes and lighting my heart with his smile. 'You will not just fly away and leave me in ignorance with just half-truths and knowledge?'

'I most certainly will not. What kind of Eagle do you take me for? I was sent here to explain you to you and to give you all the tools and knowledge to erase all your layers of ignorance, the tools you have laid down since birth, so you may connect with your true self, your soul, the place where all the answers to everything exist.'

He laughed at this, a deep splendid laugh, and then turned to me. 'Okay beautiful, you have my complete attention, so where do we start?'

Well, we shall start with understanding what is Yoga. However, I must take your leave now. We shall pick up from here next time we meet.'

With that, I turned to him and bowed to the soul within us both. I then hoped off the cliff and gave him my boldest, most elegant salutation and landed back beside him to wish him goodbye."

2

Human Meets Yoga

As I launched off his shoulder and into freedom, I heard Corey shout after me: "Wait! Come back! Give me just five more minutes of your time. I have always understood Yoga to be an exercise. If you leave me now, my mind will have a meltdown from trying to understand how an exercise can remove the power of my conditioned mind and plug me into the Universe. I mean, really, if an exercise can do that, why not just play football to reach enlightenment?"

I laughed out loud at the absurdity that had erupted from his mouth. Yoga an exercise. How did humans manage to take everything mystical and transform it into something so base, so monetary? I flew back, landed a little closer to him, and looked into his crystal blue eyes that lay on his luminous, white skin.

"Mmmmm ... where do we start? Well, let me first tell you this. The story I am going to tell you will be the story of Yoga. It is the oldest and most ancient discipline in the world. It seeks to remove the power and influence of the conditioned mind and all the layers that make up your human form, so in the silence you may connect to your pure consciousness, the *atman*.

It is a story which provides awareness about your thoughts, actions, and behaviours as judgements, criticisms, or negativities. You will need to be open-minded, so you may begin to understand yourself and the world in which you live in. Please know, Human, that all of us in nature loves every single one of your species because we see the light and goodness in all of you. Never forget that as we move through this story: Yoga seeks to show you what all of us in nature see in you, absolute love and goodness.

Across all the religions and disciplines in the world, there is a consensus that there is a soul, which in some religions is referred to as spirit. There exists also a greater being, referred to by some as God, by others as Universe, Brahman, Allah, and so forth. Here, we refer to that all-encompassing entity as universal consciousness (*purusha*). In some religions, there is also an intermediary between the two. For the purpose of our conversation, *atman* is the individual consciousness and will henceforth be referred to as the soul or spirit. Know that each soul has its own essence. It carries all the data of your incarnations before you entered the human form and all the accumulated data it will accrue on its journey forward after this form. You are, in fact, immortal, Corey.

You humans are made up of several complex parts. First, there is the soul, pure consciousness. Then there is the animal brain, which seeks to ensure your survival. I mean literal survival here, not need an iPhone and a big car survival. Above that sits your emotional and thinking brains that are constantly seeking to satisfy themselves. Then there is your body and all the layers that influence it.

The mind-body complex are part of matter that make up your entire human form, a form, you will remember, that holds all five elements, each influenced by the three *gunas* (forces) tied to it. A form that is impermanent, constantly shifting and changing as it strives to find balance. But rarely succeeding because of the lives you have embroiled yourselves in and your attachment to your human form.

In removing your entanglement with and attachment to your natural form, you can learn to live above the impermanence of nature, your nature, to find peace and joy amid chaos. You can also learn to live your true purpose, to connect to the infinite possibilities that exist for you, and to make the impossible, possible.

When a city is abandoned, notice how nature, by its own means, envelops it. It is the same with humans. If you don't learn to live above your nature, it will envelop you and take you on a emotional roller coaster ride, constantly moving you between action, tranquility, and destruction. Yoga, therefore, is the journey to learn how to enjoy life and experience it but not attach to it. It is the human attachment to an impermanent nature that is the root of all your sufferings. But don't look so confused. Remember that when you see the whole puzzle, with the knowledge of all its parts, clarity shall arrive."

"Yes," Corey the human let out a large sigh and pondered on what I had told him so far. "I most definitely will be needing more information, especially about the layers of the mind. Because I can tell you, there have been so many instances when this mind has led me and so many others to suffering, heartache, fear, joy, and love all in one week and sometimes even in one day. For some of us, it has given rise to the desire to just check out of life and dive into death."

"We have time, Corey, but you must be patient and listen to the whole story with an open mind and without wearing the various coloured glasses of white, man, father, son, brother, culture, work and all the multitude of filters through which you see the world. If you do, then I promise you that at the end of this story you will experience magic. But please know, Corey, that the story told here will also be told from such other perspectives as western and Chinese medicine, so you may know that the story I tell you is a truth."

"I'd say that sitting here with you, the most beautiful Eagle I have laid my eyes on, I am already experiencing magic. But what exactly do you mean by my 'coloured glasses'?"

"Ahh yes. Perspective and its power to arrive at self-awareness. That is for another conversation, but for now let's talk Yoga.

Yoga, my new friend, is NOT an exercise. It is a way of life, a pathway to regaining your connection to everything. I say this because, of course, you humans, like us are born with all the knowledge you need: you are not alone, you are loved and deeply connected to the Universe, you have superhero powers of telepathy, teleportation, etc. But unlike us, as you grow from birth, your subconsciousness is fed a vast array of half truths and illusions from society, media, family, friends, partners, etc. As this happens, your ignorance expands and slowly pollutes the ocean that is your mind such that the innate knowledge that sits in your soul is buried. It is this lack of knowledge about your true self that is the source of all your pain. The study of Yoga is therefore the gaining of all the knowledge to know how to erase all your learned ignorance. The study of Yoga teaches you how to quiet, purify, and control the conditioned mind, so you are able to see the reflection of your soul in it."

I could see the light growing in his eyes not only at the thought of living a life of peace and harmony with everything and engaging in violence only for literal survival, but also at the thought of being able to maybe, just maybe, grow a relationship between us, which Wind had started and only magic could sustain.

"So, what happened next?" asked the line of ants that had appeared from nowhere and taken up a whole limb. "I hope you don't mind, but Wind has been spreading the word that you are telling the story of Yoga."

"Not at all," I replied. "It is a fascinating story and one I hope that you will spread to all the humans that infringe on your life every single day. This is if you are unlucky enough to have them in your space."

"Move along, Eagle," yawned Leopard. "You know I must get 13 hours of sleep before it is time for me to seek my meal."

"Yes, my friend. I know that I am stretching the boundaries of your waking hours, so I will finish with what I left the human with.

'There are several limbs that make up the body of Yoga, all which I will, in time, describe to you in detail from the cosmic all the way down to your cells. These limbs and the trunk that

ID ACADEMY UK

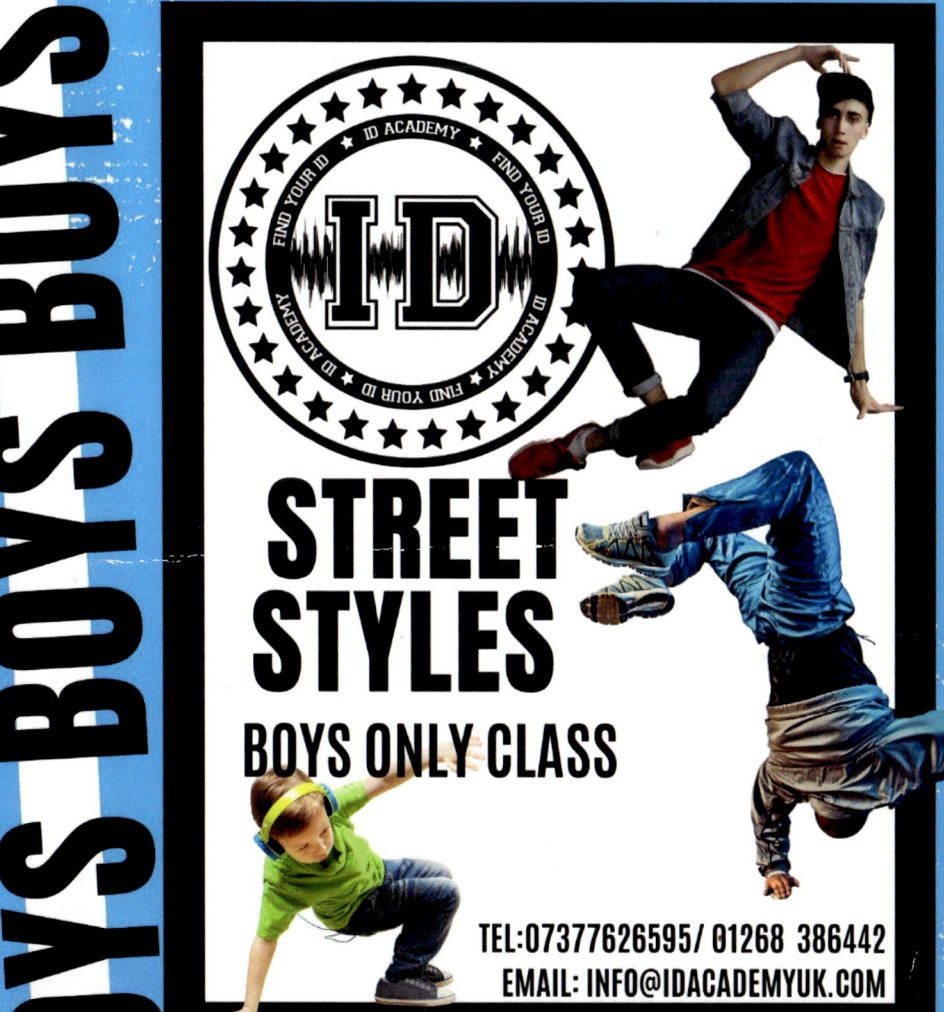

BOYS BOYS BOYS BOYS BOYS BOYS

STREET STYLES
BOYS ONLY CLASS

TEL: 07377626595 / 01268 386442
EMAIL: INFO@IDACADEMYUK.COM

TUESDAYS 6PM-7PM

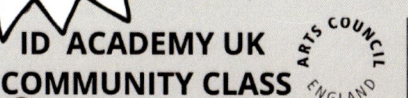

£3.00 per class

ID ACADEMY UK COMMUNITY CLASS

Supported using public funding by
ARTS COUNCIL ENGLAND

make up Yoga were codified by Patanjali, the master coder of his time, into the Yoga *sutras*. This information was passed down to the seven *rishis* (or sages) as they sat on the banks of lake Kantisarovar in the Himalayas by Adi yogi over five thousand years ago. It is a discipline that is believed to have risen from the Universe long before the first religions or belief systems.

These seven sages then traveled across the planet, which is why there are Yoga principles in every religion and ancient culture around the globe. But it is in India that the yogic system expressed itself the loudest. Corey, I know you are a religious man, so let me get this out of the way now. The greatest divide you humans have created among yourselves has been around religion. Hinduism is steeped in Yoga, but Yoga is not Hinduism. It is a discipline that anyone, from any category, can practise. You can be a part of any religion, caste, race, nationality, gender, etc., and still follow the journey of Yoga because its main goal is to reconnect you with your true self and then to the universal consciousness. All Yoga asks of you is to take up the tools it offers, practise them, and witness their truth for yourself.

Yoga has no quarrel with religion or any other discipline in the world today as they are all paths to the same destination. Each religion, each discipline should be viewed as exactly that, a path to destination enlightenment. The journey is a personal one, so it does not matter what path your partners, friends, or co-workers are on; if they are on a path to self-knowledge that should be enough. Because what ties all of us to each other, Corey, is the consciousness and love that lives in all of us. Don't let anyone tell you that humans are evil. At your core, when you move past all the layers that define the human form, you are all good. You have just forgotten it.

Yoga needs no temple, no altar, no costume, nor a surrender to anyone or anything. Yoga asks only that you surrender to the Universal consciousness that is connected to you via your soul. It asks that you learn to love you, a self love that is different from a selfish love. Through self-love, what grows is a desire to love all living beings and give selflessly. You, Corey, and no one else are the source of your happiness, of peace and calmness, and the definer of your reality.

At its simplest level, there are eight limbs that make up the tree of Yoga. The first limbs are *yamas* and *niyamas*, the ethical guidelines on how to interact and behave with others and the world you find yourselves inhabitants of. By following these, you move through your life with joy and calmness as they serve to purify your mind., and it is only in a pure, clean mind that you can see the reflection of your soul.

Then there are the *asanas* (or poses), the physical practise of Yoga. *Asanas* connect you with your body and begin the process of unravelling blocked energy channels within you. They also strengthen and stretch your body, so it no longer acts as an impediment to sitting in meditation.

After that there is breathing, that thing so many of you humans take for granted and don´t even do properly either because your body is so hunched up that it blocks your diaphragm from expanding and using the full capacity of your lungs or because you are just too lazy to exercise the lung muscle. Which is shocking when you think that without breath your form would die. But I digress, the limb of breathing is more than just about influencing your breath. It is also about unblocking and moving your energy as well as calming your *gunas* to bring you back into homeostasis.'"

I turned to the growing clan and sighed in exasperation. "I really don't get it. How is it that humans spend hours on their hair, their bodies, their looks, phones, TV, work, and barely minutes on their breath, the thing that keeps their body alive?"

To this, the whole posse that had gathered burst out in laughter and nodded in agreement.

Yoga, Where the Impossible Meets the Possible

"I know, I know, Leopard. I am nearly at the end of today's story time. Where was I, ummm, yes, of course, breathing. I continued to tell him the following:

'For you humans, Corey, there are numerous breathing techniques to move, shift, and unblock trapped energy within your bodies. Each *pranayama*, as it is known in Yoga, not only ignites and widens the energetic magnetic field that exists around each of you, but also serves to lift your electrical brain waves to gamma, the highest frequency where that connection to the information in the infinite space is made possible.

The next limb is the process of withdrawing from your senses, so you can engage in awareness as a means of observing all the conditionings of the mind that form the basis of **ME**, your personality. This process leads ultimately to you connecting to your true self, known as your **I,** your soul. By learning to concentrate deeply on one thing, as opposed to superficially on several things, you can move into meditation with ease. Then there is meditation, the connector to the infinite space, so that you may finally merge and become one with the Universe, as opposed to living in the belief that you are separate from it.

To summarise, let me simplify all eight limbs for you. There are *yamas*, i.e., restraints and abstinence; *niyamas*, i.e., observances and training; *asanas*, i.e., gaining mastery over meditative postures; *pranayama*, i.e., the control over energy through the regulation and expansion of breath; *pratyahara*, i.e., the withdrawal from satisfying your desires and senses externally by turning the senses inwards; *dharana*, i.e., concentration of the mind on one thing; *dhyana*, i.e., meditation through effortless concentration; and lastly, *samadhi*, contemplation and then absorption into the object of meditation so that the observer and the observed unite into a superconscious state.'

And then I ended with this, just to plant a seed of thought into his subconscious:

'Did you know, Corey, that when you humans clear cut rainforests, destroy habitats, and kill animals, you are, in fact, killing yourselves, literally? Because you are a part of the whole ecosystem; you too are nature. Thought of another way, the energetic earth is one body with two arms, two legs, a head, and, well, you get the drift. And you the human are one of the legs, Ocean another, Forest an arm, and so forth. When you cut down a part of nature, which you see yourself as separate from, you are cutting off parts of a body of which you are a part. Basically, you are cutting your own arms off. And if we go a step further, Earth itself is part of a large cosmic body also comprised of several body parts in the form of planets, stars, black holes, etc. When you destroy nature, it destroys the Earth, which is then cutting off a body part of the planetary system. Are you beginning to see just how your one human species is bringing the entire Universe into imbalance? Yet when you wake up, your largest problem is how much money you have, how your hair looks, what is trending on social media, what are others thinking of you, etc. So, tell me, Corey, are all of you humans just plain ol' insane, crazy, or just deeply unaware?'

I could see smoke coming out of his head and his mind moving and shifting. Somewhere in the recess of his conditioned mind, I saw a tiny light appear. Of course, I wanted to fly to the Moon and back in excitement, but I contained myself. I knew for that light to grow, for the connection to be made and for suffering to no longer have power, it was a long journey and hard work. It was one thing for me to give him the tools, it was another for him to pick them up and begin to use them. Understanding there was no app, 31-day program, one week retreat, or Fitbit watch that would get him to destination enlightenment. Only doing the work every day would get him there.

As I finished my Eagle Yoga monologue, Corey placed his hand on my wing and whispered, 'Thank you for crawling into my mind and burying yourself in my soul. I want what you have, unwavering belief in the connection to everything. My journey as a human has been hard, filled with pain, fear, suffering, and acts of love that feel nothing like what love should feel like. I know you must go now, but tell me, when can we meet again? I would like to begin this magical journey of Yoga about which you speak so passionately.'

I shivered, I did, from the feel of him on my wings. If I could have kissed him with my beak without eating his mouth, I would have, but instead I turned to him and spoke.

'Only when the Moon is full or new do all the elements conspire to allow nature, of which you are a part, to communicate with the human. If you follow the cliff to where Forest meets Ocean, you will find an enormous baobab tree. Meet me there next new moon, and it is there that we will continue this story.'"

"You what?! You told him to come here, to this sacred place? Have you lost your beak?!" stuttered Snake, who had dropped in from the highest of Baobab's limbs.

"Hold on there, Snake," bellowed Baobab. "You forget: he is one of us, and the sooner he knows that the better, before the humans take their machines and kill us all off, and themselves in the process. Is it not more advisable that he learns and understands that connection through us who live in that connection every moment of our lives?"

"True be that. I am sorry. I get a little slithery around humans. They always look at me as if I were some evil being sent to cause them harm, even though I have no interest in them at all. Man, that box of theirs that they stare at for hours on end is a brainwash box that puts crazy illusionary ideas in their heads."

For a moment we all sat, hung, swung, and flowed in silence, thinking of that black screen that spewed out lies, gossip, and half truths. The box that seemed to mesmerize the human and then guide, influence, and define their behaviours, all without them knowing what it was doing. Little did they know that the workings of their own brain and mind and how everything they listened to and watched was recorded in their hippocampus hard drive, their subconscious.

"What did he say? Is he going to come?" fluttered Butterfly back and forth.

"He is," I smiled. "And get this, he hugged me before he left, and I rubbed my wings all over him, trying to leave as much of my scent on him before he walked away."

I giggled, remembering the twinkle in his eyes.

"Then I gently lay my wing upon his heart and said, 'May you be well until we meet again. May you know that you are not your mind, your thoughts, or your emotions. May every word, action, and behaviour that rises from you between now and when we meet again rise from a place of love and never from a place of fear. And may you wake up every day grateful for the opportunity to experience this magnificent Universe in a human form.'"

"Fabulous," smiled Baobab. "Now, kindly remove yourselves from my 3000-year-old limbs and go off on your merry way. We shall meet at the new moon and see if the human truly seeks change. If he does, he will return."

With that we all leapt, flew, and jumped off Baobab. We wished each other well on our journeys and promised to meet again at new moon.

3

Nature Welcomes the Human

At the new moon, we once again congregated on and around Baobab. We seemed to have grown in numbers as word had spread, and nearly all of nature was curious to understand human behaviours. That species in one way or another was affecting all of us, mostly in a negative way.

Not one of us feared that the human, if he dared to engage in change and show up, would be overwhelmed by such a diverse gathering of friends. At some point, we had all witnessed humans ignore us unless they were seeking to irradiate or move us for their benefit. They walked around completely unaware of their present and, hence, their surroundings. Their mind was either in the past, a place that no longer existed, or in the future, a place that had yet to arrive. Consequently, they were never in their life or their present, so we, the rest of nature, for the most part remained invisible to them.

A great human thinker, Alan Watts, once said this: Most humans live in the past on events that they have not experienced directly, in other words, history, or in the past that is not here except in the form of reflective memory, or they live in the future, which is also not here except in the imagined form of anticipation. These humans thus live in an impoverished present best represented by a hair-line cross point between the past and the future. Ever notice how on a watch the present is a tiny, hairline hand? This is because humans see the present as boring and humdrum. They are completely unaware of all the life that surrounds them. They do not know how to be alive by being present in the richness of the Universe and all its manifestations.

We began to find our places as peace descended upon us. We then settled into each others' energy and waited calmly. Each of us was enjoying the different frequencies that we emitted, the warmth of Sun, the history of Baobab, and the power of Ocean.

Nature Welcomes the Human

"Nature," I began, "before the human arrives, which I have no doubt he will, I wanted to say something to all of you. I know we have all had negative experiences with humans and are confused by that species. However, let us always remember that there are those among them where good has risen to the surface. Humans who speak to the Universe and to us and who seek to push their species into the light. We know that at the core of every single human there is good as the creator of all lives in all of us.

There is no judgement or arrogance in the story we are about to tell, just a desire to raise awareness in the human of the difference between the functioning of their form and that of their soul. As it is their form that creates suffering in them and their soul that give rise to humanity and humility in them."

I could see the nods, the wobbles, and the gentle sway of yeses rise all around me.

"I see him. I see him. Well, I think it is him as I have never met him before, but he is a handsome bugger. I assume it is him," Orangutan, swinging back and forth in somersaults, sang out loud from the top branch of Baobab.

I could feel the excitement move as a wave. I lifted my wings and ascended toward the sky. It was him indeed. Carrying his muscles with confidence and his heart out front, he was whistling a happy tune and built like a rock. Yet he had felt soft when I had touched him, and his bald head was perfectly shaped. I could feel the sway in this hips that matched the tune from his mouth. That is, until he reached the tree and stopped dead in his tracks.

I landed gently on his shoulder, and he looked at me with the most bewildered look on his face. He opened his mouth, and all that was released was air. I could already hear his words.

"Eagle, there are hundreds of animals here, I, ahhh, I," he stuttered. "I thought it would be only you and me."

I could hear giggles erupting all around me and thought it best I explain their laughter before it shot him right back out into his human heavy world.

"Weeeeelll, here's the thing. It seems that there are many of us who seek to understand the human. When word got out I was telling the story of Yoga and its understanding of the Human, they all showed up. Or they felt the need to chaperone me in case you get any funny ideas of kidnapping me and turning me into some experiment. Don´t think I did not notice the gun on you the first time we met."

At this, Corey burst out into the largest laughter I imagined could come out of a human mouth and did not stop for minutes. When he finally found his normal, uninfluenced, autonomous breath, he turned to me.

"I am a lawman of the government type, but for humans only. We don´t directly protect other species, so you are safe with me. And really, if I were to kidnap you, it would not be for an experiment," he winked at me.

"Whaat?" Hawk flew into the air and landed on Corey's shoulder. "You would kidnap her to eat her!"

"No no no. That is not what I meant, what I meant was......."

"Yesss?" the living Baobab and all the visitors asked in unison.

I could see the red rising from his feet all the way up to his head. I knew I could rescue him here, but I was curious as to how he would rescue himself.

"It's just that she is so beautiful and ... and well."

"Okay, let's give the human a break, shall we and instead give him a proper greeting?"

At once, every single one of us, from trees to Ocean to animals and plants turned toward him and presented him with their own salutations. It was a cacophony of bows, twists, forward bends, back bends, and inversions. I don't believe he had ever witnessed such beauty and synchronicity. I watched his face transform into a look of wonder. Once we had all finished our salutations and settled down, I invited the Human to climb upon Baobab and sit on the lowest limb, which was as thick as a bed. I then settled down beside him.

He smiled at me, and I felt his energy shift to a place of calmness. "I have thought about you much since we last met. At our last meeting, you talked a lot about the conditioned mind. I was hoping we could maybe start there."

I felt a flutter move through me, flattered that he had listened to every word we had exchanged.

"Eagle, do you mind if I explain this one to him? After all, as an Orangutan, my brain is closest to his," asked Orangutan as she lowered herself onto our branch, lay down, and boldly placed her head on the human's lap.

At this, Corey smiled at me and shrugged his shoulders. "I am surrendering here to your wisdom and your guidance. I hold no resistance, so if this hairy monkey with her wide eyes and beautiful face wants to tell me a part of this story, I have no problem. All I ask is that you remain perched beside me as she does."

Thank you, Universe, for not giving me the ability to blush. If you had, I would have turned into a whole different colour than the white, brown, and black that dominated me with a tinge of yellow. "Of course I will, and yes, Orangutan is really the best one to explain this concept to you. But first, there is something I need you to do for me to bring you fully into the present moment, which is your life."

"Anything," he replied. "All you have to do is ask."

"Grab each of your butt cheeks and pull them to the side and back, so you are sitting on your sitting bones. The last thing I want is for you to leave here with a pain in your back."

At this request, he looked at me funny, but he decided to humour me as he spied Leopard lounging and smiling with joy above him. I watched Corey's brain flirt with all the animal shows he'd watched on the black box leading him to interpret that smile as hunger. Ahhh, how much of the world's suffering stems from misunderstanding.

"Now close your eyes, lift the crown of your head up toward Sky, and ground your sitting bones into Baobab while lengthening your spine and opening your chest. Begin to be aware of all nature's elements surrounding you: the sound of a hundred animals breathing that same air as you; the feel of the wind moving through you; the power of Ocean filling your ears. Sense the trees swaying and smell the blossoming of hundreds of flowers. Feel the warmth of Sun, the security of Sky, the creativity of the clouds, and be grounded by Earth below you. Know that their energy is connected to yours and not separate from it. Allow all of nature's energy to move through you and lift your own energy to a place of gratitude.

Now gently drop out of your thinking mind and into your feeling body. Acknowledge and accept what you are feeling at this very moment without judgment or attachment Understand that emotions are indicators of where you are stuck, where your energy is blocked.

Now shift your awareness to your breath. Feel how your body moves with each inhale and exhale. Does your breath rise from your chest or your belly? Is it fast or slow? Constant or erratic? What is your breath telling you about you? For breath reflects the movements occurring within you. When you are in fear, the breath starts and ends in your chest and is fast and erratic. When you are calm, the breath is slow and starts from your belly. Just take a moment to observe you.

Now gently begin to influence your breath. As you inhale, begin to expand your belly gently. Then feel your chest move as your ribs move out and up, filling your underarms, your throat, and your head with fresh oxygen and energy. Pause for just a moment, holding your breath in relaxation, storing all the energy you have just inhaled into your brain or solar plexus. Now slowly exhale and feel your ribs move down and in and your belly in and up. With each inhale, feel your diaphragm lower and massage all your organs. With each exhale, feel your diaphragm gently lift and squeeze your calming parasympathetic Vagus nerve, so it will release a substance that slows down your heart. Now take a moment to just follow your breath to find the top of your inhale and finish your exhale. With each exhale, gently step out of your boxes, your stereotypes, your roles, your labels, and just be present with us on this tree.

Life is only this moment, this inhale, this exhale, so be present in your life. Be present with us. Now open your heart to the knowledge and truths we will share with you today and in the days to follow such that, in time, what lays in front of you in this moment called life looks nothing like what lay behind you. Slowly rub your hands together, place them over your eyes, and take a big sigh. On your next exhale, lower your hands and move yourself from behind the veil of darkness and into the light that shines all around you."

With that Corey slowly lowered his hands, opened his eyes, and looked around him, seeing and feeling us for the first time. It was like watching a child that had yet to be ruined by ignorance. We all watched the smile of wonder slowly spread across his face. He was speechless, but that was just fine for all of us. We could all feel and read his energy, an energy that had slowly shifted from chaos to complete calmness.

"So, this is what it means to be present with awareness," he whispered, still in awe of all that he was feeling. "To live in the present by connecting to all the wonders that surround me."

"Yes, Corey," sang all the flowers that had blossomed in that moment. "Every single day, we speak to you humans. We offer healing, calmness, colour, and so many different vibrations, but so many of you walk right by us and never connect. You are either on a phone, staring at the perceived lives of others, or subconsciously moving through the hundreds of habits you have accumulated without even knowing it. Thereby allowing your mind to be anywhere but in the present. Your habits ensure you no longer have to be aware of how to walk, what route to take to work, or when to cross the road. No, you are on autopilot, so your mind can be as far away from your present, and hence your life, as possible."

"Okay, okay," trumpeted the elephants who had just arrived. "Let's give Corey a break, shall we? The poor guy is here representing all of humanity and is probably adjusting to being a minority in a world where he, the human, is normally the majority. Besides, I think it is safe to say that he is fully present as he sits on a tree next to an Eagle with Orangutan's head on his lap and an elephant coming to his defense.

Hello, Corey. We are pleased to have you here, us elephants especially as we too would like to share our energy, our emotions, and our joy with you. We are not so different from the human."

At this, we all watched Corey wonder what on Earth he shared with an elephant, for it was not the size of their trunks. Suddenly giggles spread like wildfire, and baby monkeys started to fall off the tree and onto the ground. They could no longer hold on so tickled where they by the human's thought process.

"No, Corey, it is not our trunks," came the deep rumbling voice of the largest elephant. "It is how we mourn the loss of our dead and love our living, but we shall hold that conversation for another moon, shall we?"

Corey just nodded, unable to conjure up any sound as he watched the elephants find their place near the water. For a moment, we felt Corey sink into deep thought, and we allowed him the space and love to dwell there.

Nature Welcomes the Human

"You know, I was married for a very long time to someone who treated me very poorly. It was like being married to a yoyo. Sometimes she showered me in love. Other times she threw me into the pit of suffering and unkindness. So much so that as I sit here today I no longer trust words of love or believe myself to be worthy of love. I have built walls inside of me from the experiences of my past such that no one may ever hurt me again. In a way, you are 100% correct. I always step forth into my present and my future with all the walls, boundaries, and memories of my past." He looked at me as if a tiny firecracker had exploded in his head.

"I really am limiting my present and hence my future, aren´t I? It will just keep looking like my past, and there is a good chance I will never experience a great love for myself the way you all sit so comfortably in self-love and in love for each other."

We all nodded in unison, and I felt his sadness wash over me. He then turned and stared deep into my eyes. "How do I erase this past from my mind and step forth to live as you all do, in the present fully without effort and always moving from a place of love and never from fear? I may be a human, but never have I felt such an enormous energy of love as I do sitting here in this moment."

"Well that my handso, I mean, Corey, is what the story of Yoga is all about. Love. Love for yourself, for the Universe within you and all around you, for all living beings. Now I have been told by Sun that she is on a timer, so we best begin before she sets."

Orangutan straightened herself up and began to pace up and down and all-around Baobab until finally she came back to where Corey sat and began:

"I think we need to move away from the laws of the Universe for a moment and shift to the human mind. So, let's talk biology first, shall we? At the base of the human brain is the brain stem, also known as the mammalian brain, because yes, it is the oldest part of your brain and the part that most resembles ours."

Here the Orangutan puffed out her chest as if she alone had been responsible for the creation of the animal brain. "It is your instinctual brain and the throne of your autonomous nervous system (ANS), your respiratory system, your digestion system, your heartbeat, and so forth. These are all systems you cannot control but over which you can exert influence.

This part of the brain is also known as your instinctual survival brain because its origins go back to a time when you needed it to hunt, procreate, sleep, and preserve your species. When you live in this part of the brain, you react without thought and automatically behave in a way that seeks survival. However, the problem with that in today's human world is that the benchmark and definition of survival and security has changed. For you humans, survival has become something elusive, constantly shifting, and never truly attainable. Examples of this are..."

"Oo! Wait. I know," howled Wolf. "I have heard these phrases from them when they are camping in the mountain.

'I need that job and that promotion;'

'I need to be with someone;'

'I need to make more money;'

'I need a car, and I need a phone;'

'I need to look a certain way.'

Understand that the word *need* means that without that item, the person in question will not be able to survive."

"Okay. I get your point, Wolf," laughed Corey. "There is a possibility that we Humans may have completely lost touch with what it means to survive." Before he could say anything else, Orangutans face appeared swinging from side to side before his.

"Now Corey, on top of the brain stem is the next level of your brain, the limbic brain, also know as your emotional brain. It is the place where you store all incoming data and the emotions you attach to them and where your hard drive sits with your memories and your emotions. Basically, it is the soap opera part of your brain."

In one big swing, Orangutan swung off the branch and landed on the other side of Corey. "The last layer of your brain, well, there are more areas, but for our purpose we only focus on these three main areas, is the frontal cortex. This is the thinking, analytical part of the human brain that sadly is very underused in the human for purposes of happiness and joy."

"I think we need to stop there for today," I said as I flew onto Orangutan's head. "I know we were supposed to start with the mind, but sometimes things just don't work out as planned. And that is okay. That is the nature of life. In fact, before we even get to the mind, we need to understand what consciousness is because this is the foundation of everything and not a small topic."

I turned to Corey. "We will get to the mind, I promise. This story is huge, and sometimes it will flow down different tributaries. But by the end they will all lead us to the soul. Do you want me to walk you back to the road? You can carry me on your shoulder, if you don't mind."

"Not at all," he blushed. "I would love nothing more than to carry you with me everywhere."

At that, he swung off the tree, landed squarely on his feet, and turned to the orchestra of nature's beauties. He then bent down and touched Earth.

"Thank you for reminding me that I am you and you are me, that I am nature, and that these magnificent creatures are not separate from me but deeply connected to me. As I move through these days waiting for the next rising full moon, I shall make every effort to acknowledge all of nature that appears around me every day, to feel it, listen to it, see it, be apart of it, and respect it. It will make the effort of being present so much easier because I will be present with all of you."

With that, we all moved through our salutations once more and bid him farewell. I landed gently on his shoulder, and he began to walk. At first, we sat in a comfortable silence, just listening and feeling the other.

"Do you think us meeting was a coincidence or something that was meant to be?" he asked softly.

"There is no such thing as chance," I replied. "Every single effect has a cause that is governed by the laws of the Universe, of which we are a product. Therefore, our meeting was not by chance, but a direct result of a cause or a series of causes that can go as far back as our past lives. Everything that is happening now between us has a relationship to that which came before it. We were destined to meet. I was sent to you not only to give you the tools to move your soul forward, but also to teach you what pure love looks like, not the romantic love that you humans peddle to each other all the time."

"Love," he rolled it on his tongue, tasting it as if it were his first time.

"Yes, Love. Love as the Universe has for everything. Love as light. Love without judgement, expectations, or boundaries. I know you think it impossible for such a love to exist between you and I, but by the time I finish this story, you will see that nothing is impossible."

I could feel his doubt, his fears, and see his walls, but they did not deter me. I knew the power of Yoga just as I knew the power of Love: because it to had influenced my journey into an Eagle.

He continued to walk in silence, afraid of what he might say. When we came to the place where we could go no further, I flew off his shoulder onto a rock and waited.

"Is it strange that I have these feelings for you that stir from a place that I do not know? And a mind that is telling me that we are too different, from different worlds, conflicting colours, cultures, backgrounds, and to entertain such thoughts is insanity?"

"It is not strange at all; it is the way your human mind has been conditioned to see this world, to always see separation and difference because you spend a vast amount of your lives focusing on the external. But be patient and, in time, all those boxes you or others have put you in will begin to disappear, as will this form that you see as a barrier between us. It's okay. You can run your hands over my feathers."

"How did you know I was thinking that?" he asked surprised. But in my silence, he remembered all he had been told thus far. His face turned into awareness as he understood that I could read the information held in his energy. He gently reached out and lay his hands on the back of my neck. It was as if I had been hit by lightning. In that one touch, I felt not only warmth and electricity run through my entire being, but also his fears of what he was feeling.

Time stopped and for what seemed like decades but was mere moments, we stood like that. Then he slowly removed his hand and smiled. "I will see you at the next full moon." And with that, he turned around and went back to his world where everything was perceived as separate from everything else.

4

Ocean Explains Consciousness

"I hope he got my message. I used good ol' fashioned telepathy during my meditation last night to tell Corey to come as the moon was rising," I said as I landed on Baobab and greeted the new arrivals.

"Hahahahha!" screeched hyenas who had arrived the day before, eager to join the gathering and learn more about the Humans who had portrayed them as scavengers instead of cute and cuddly like Panda who sat beside them chewing on a bamboo shoot.

"Telepathy? You know most humans don´t believe in that? Which is a little surprising as they never question a paper coming out of a fax machine with a message from a million miles away or the transmission of images via Wi-Fi."

"I hear you, scavenger," giggled Panda, playing lovingly with Hyena. "Did you know that if you throw a stone into a pool of water, it produces a ripple of waves traveling outward just as the light from a candle gives rise to waves of ethereal vibrations moving out in all directions? It is the same with thoughts, good and evil, when they cross the mind of a person. It gives rise to vibrations in the *manas* (which I know Elephant is going to explain to the human), or the mental atmosphere, which then travels far and wide in all directions using ether as the vehicle to transport our thoughts just as *prana* is a vehicle for feeling and air is a vehicle for sound."

From nowhere, a large rumbling sound manifested into a vibration that shook the hundreds of animals that had gathered on and around Baobab. What emerged from the sound were whales of every imaginable kind, rising from Ocean, splashing their love all over us.

"We heard your thoughts, Eagle," spoke the smallest whale among them, "because every thought you send out never dies. It goes on vibrating in every particle of the Universe, which is how we heard you from halfway around the world. Sorry, it has taken us so long to get here."

With that, the whole pod of whales let out a spectacular fountain of water from their blowholes until Ocean looked as if it were dancing with the space between itself and Sky. We could hear the water sing and felt the excitement and connection between all of us.

"Thank you," I bowed to them. "It is because my thoughts are noble and forcible that they ignited a vibration in every sympathetic mind on this planet. And because you are conscious, I know my thoughts resonated with you and that you, in turn, sent out similar thoughts. In the coming weeks, I expect we shall see more of Ocean's inhabitants. We are all lucky that all our mental vibrations, no matter what our form, are in tune with each other. Humans, however, among themselves or with us, are not in tune, so misunderstanding quickly erupts between them and with the rest of nature. Then add the series of negative, lustful, jealous, hate-filled thoughts that fill their minds and block their energy channels, and it is no wonder they never really hear each other."

"And ever notice how humans often sit in sickness mentally and physically?" whispered slowly awakening Leopard. "It is because they speak so much gossip, half-truths, and lies that they have lost their connection to the power of thought. They do not understand that every single thought is conveyed to every cell in the body through the nerves such that if those thoughts are negative, filled with jealousy, anger, and hate, the cells move into a state of panic and think they are being attacked. Those cells have been raised to believe that the only time a human will move into negativity and fear is when it is being attacked.

Yoga, Where the Impossible Meets the Possible

Now if those cells stay in this state of panic due to prolonged stress and negativity they will eventually become weakened and no longer be able to perform their functions. They become inefficient. The chain reaction is that all the systems slow down as the vibration of the cells become inharmonious. What you then see is a large part of the human species feeling hopeless, low in confidence, fearful, anxious, and unhappy. It's because their life force is malfunctioning. The human cellular system was not designed to remain in a state of panic and stress. This is why the human body comes with a calming as well as an active flight or flight system."

At this moment, a group of butterflies landed all over Leopard and in a beautiful melody sang, "it is so magical that our thoughts are pure and full of light, that our brain is simple, but our consciousness enormous."

"You got that right," rolled the rocks in unison at the edge of Ocean. "Hey Eagle, did you explain to Human that thought is the greatest force on earth and the most powerful weapon of the Yogi? For is it not so, Eagle, that thought is the primal force behind the origin of all creation?"

"You are correct in your knowledge," I replied flying around the gathered representatives of nature. I could feel the energy of the Human making his way to me. "The genesis of the entire phenomenal creation we know as the Universe and Earth's place within it began as a single thought that arose in the cosmic mind. Therefore, the world is the primal idea made manifest. This first thought became manifested as a vibration issuing from the Eternal Stillness of the Divine Essence, which I explained is *purusha,* the universal consciousness. This vibration is nothing like the rapid oscillation back-and-forth of physical particles. It is something infinitely more subtle, so subtle as to be inconceivable to the normal human mind. But let me reassure you that all forces, forms, and thoughts are ultimately resolvable into a state of pure vibration. Hence why the words we use are so important; it is believed that each word carries a vibration that moves beyond us, resonates, and affects every living thing. Thoughts, like *gunas*, are a force that can affect matter positively or negatively."

At that moment as we all stilled to ponder each others' thoughts, Moon began to rise. It presented itself as luminous with a rainbow of circular energy radiating around it.

"Good evening," arrived the deep voice of Moon that resonated over each one of us like a slow, deep massage. "It is a glorious gift to see all of you in one place on one wavelength. You have no idea how long I have waited for this moment. For decades I have watched humans slowly decimate my soul mate, Earth, feeling her pain and her torment. Until they decided to land on me and leave bits of their litter on me as well. Finally, I will have the opportunity to learn about humans, the species that spend their energy traveling into space instead of healing Earth and each other. The faster humans can understand themselves, the better because it may just save the rest of us rotating up here from their invasion."

"Uuuhuh. Uhhunn," grunted my buddy Orangutan, who was now hanging upside down in front of me and avoiding me poking her eyes out with my beak.

"He is arriving," Moon silenced us in his whisper. "Eagle go get your Human and guide him safely to us. Try not to smother him with the endless love and light that flows forth from you; most humans are not ready for such radiance. They do not trust it as love in their world has often been used to harm, manipulate, and destroy; it opens them up and makes them vulnerable. And it is this vulnerability and fear of pain that keeps them sitting closed off inside the walls of fear instead."

I nodded my head to Moon and flew off to meet Corey. I was sure they could all hear my heart beating loud and fast as if it wanted my head to explode so it might have the room it sought to somersault and jump and fill all the space around me., I could hear him humming before I saw him. For a moment, I hovered above him to feel his joy.

"I know you are up there. I feel you," he said without looking up.

"Hello, Corey. It is nice to see you again." I smiled as I landed on his broad shoulders. We chatted lightly until he reached the edge of Ocean and his mouth fell open. Across Ocean and in the silhouette of Moon, lay dozens of whales on their backs, basking in the love of Moon. He then slowly turned to me and stuttered, "iiissss, arree those, whhh whhhalles?"

"Yes, Corey, they are," swooned Baobab. "It would seem your species has touched nearly all of us in such a way that has left us bamboozled about your kind. But you are safe with us. Eagle has vouched for you, and her word is enough for us. Please climb up and have a seat. Hawk, move your feathered bottom a little, would you, to make room for Corey?"

"Sure. Sure, but first I have a question. Who are you, Corey?" asked Hawk scrutinizing him softly.

At this Corey stopped and took a moment to compile his answer. "Well, I am a law enforcement agent, a Christian, a black belt in jitsu, I am American..."

"Whoooo there, Human" said Panda as it padded over to Corey and stood beside him. "You are telling us all the things you do and the roles you play but not who you are."

With this, the Human's face took on the very familiar look of confusion, and he just stared at Panda as if it were senseless.

"Don't give him a hard time," rose the deep voice of Ocean, causing all the whales to roll over and dive down into the belly of Ocean, tickling it on the way down. "He knows not what you mean by that question. Corey, it is fine. Ignore Panda. Hop up onto Baobab, and we will start today's journey into the human mind with some basics."

Ocean Explains Consciousness

Corey climbed up the tree and sat with Leopard on one side, me on the other, and Orangutan and Hawk above. All around us, hundreds of animals were either sitting, hanging, swinging, or laying on or around the majestic tree.

His gaze moved all around him until it rested on Moon.

"Well hello, Human," Moon vibrated its thoughts into Corey's mind. "Welcome and thank you for being open to seeing yourself from our perspective, the perspective of the Universe. I know it is hard to believe there is a reality that is so very different from the one you perceive. I know most humans think reality is what they see and do not understand that all reality is merely perception. Here, let me make this a little easier for you to understand."

And, just like that, dropped a tire from out of Sky.

"What do you see, Butterfly?" asked Ocean.

"Well, umm, yaa, not sure. It looks like a strange sort of tree, with a hole in it, where I could possibly lay my head."

"And you, Hyena, what do you see?"

"Food, of course, and if you don't mind, I would be pleased to take a bite out of it."

"Just hold on there, Hyena. You cannot eat the object of the lesson in the middle of the lesson. Now Corey, what do you see?"

Corey looked up at Moon with the most confused face he could muster and mumbled as if he were not too sure of his answer anymore, "A tire that belongs on a car."

The entire posse of nature laughed until they had to stop to catch their breath.

"Okay, settle down, wild things. Corey, what you call a 'tire' is matter. All matter is made up of particles that are constantly moving, and all particles have energy. The amount of energy varies depending on the form of the matter. This tire, as you call it, is slow vibrating molecules that have taken on a shape that you perceive as a tire. Butterfly perceives the same thing as a home, and forever hungry Hyena perceives it as food.

If the object were, in fact, a tire, in itself, born a tire, destined forever to be a tire, then anyone who encountered it would immediately see it as a tire; it would present itself as such. But alas, it is not. Like everything in this world, reality is merely how you perceive the energy and its forms around you. It can, in fact, be anything you want it to be.

I can see you are still a little bamboozled, so let me speak human here. Imagine an event happens and it is on the black box. If you were to access ten different channels from around the world, I can bet my gravitational connection to Earth that each one would view the same event differently. Who is right? None of them or all of them?

Tomorrow when you wake up, make a choice to take off the glasses of reality you have been wearing and put on ours. When you walk through your day, see good where once you saw bad and react with happiness where once you would react with annoyance. Remind yourself that everything is that blank screen of millions of vibrating dots and you can choose what reality you want to draw on it."

A slow smile spread over Corey's face as he began to realise not only the power he had in defining his life, rather than having it defined for him, but also that he was learning about matter from Moon.

Just then, Earth let out a massive AUM, and for a moment all our forms disappeared such that there was nothing but vibrating energy everywhere. When she finished her AUM, our forms returned. I looked over at Corey, who looked like he had seen a ghost. "Are you okay?" I whispered into his ear while also trying not to poke his brain out with my beak.

Ocean Explains Consciousness

"Ahhhh ya, I think so. That was unbelievable. I felt my body melt away as the vibration broke down my form, and I melted into peace. How did that happen?"

"The earth AUMed, which holds a frequency of 7.83 hertz. Not surprisingly, of the five brain waves that have been categorized in the human brain, alpha waves are the closest frequency to AUM. This is the state in which you, the humans, begin to move into relaxation as you shift from the conscious to the subconscious," I replied.

"I think it is time that we introduced Corey to consciousness. Don´t you think so, Ocean? I know the elephants were going to tell this story, but I believe it best fits your form," resonated Earth.

"You are correct about that, Earth. Corey, climb off Baobab and come a little closer to me. Whale, can you go to shore so that Corey may climb on your back? I want to feel him as I explain this enormous topic. Yes, Eagle. you can come as well." Ocean laughed its deep enormous laugh that created another vibration in all of us.

Corey hopped off the tree like a child filled with excitement that he was going to not only be close to a whale, but also sit on its back and have a chat with Ocean. Well, more like Ocean would chat and he would be spellbound.

A whale shark the size of a submarine emerged from Ocean and offered its back to both the human and me. He was warm, and we could feel him caress us softly with his heart. It was his way of welcoming us and conveying that we were safe with him as we were with all whales.

"Corey, before Ocean begins its tale, I think I need to make clear to you the distinctions between the mind, brain, and consciousness. Due to the limitations of language and you not being on telepathy with the Universe yet, I will try my best to explain it to you with words. The brain is an organ like any other organ in the human body. It aids and abets the mind, but in Yoga we don´t pay much attention to it. In Yoga, the main characters are the mind, which is the tool through which consciousness manifests, the human body, with its physical, mental, and emotional layers, and the Atman, the soul. Together they form the most sophisticated machine in the world through which you can experience the Universe: your consciousness. Understand?"

"I think so?" muttered Corey, who was slightly intimidated that, for all his knowledge, he was being schooled by Moon on what it meant to be in a Human form. "But I am still very unclear about this consciousness concept."

Moon´s radiance expanded as it smiled down upon the gathering. As the circles that danced around it grew, a deep calm spread across the Ocean and the Earth.

"You and most of humanity." And the Ocean, with a vibration that was as deep as it was wide began:

"All energy carries consciousness in it. Consciousness is the intelligent energy that created everything. Put another way, everything that is energy carries consciousness, but at different frequencies. It cannot be fully described with words. As it is a creator, it holds all truths. It is the cosmic intelligence that knows all. Every living thing has consciousness just as every living thing is energy, but only humans have the sophisticated mechanism to access that consciousness. Therefore, never forget that it is a privilege to be a human for only in your form can you connect with the cosmic intelligence on a more complex level."

I could see Corey's eyes light up. They reflected Ocean in the blueness that never seized to amaze me. He had never really thought of being human as a privilege before, and I could sense a tiny shift in the way he saw himself.

Ocean Explains Consciousness

"Whoa. Hold on, Ocean" purred Lion who sat majestically at the edge of Ocean. His mane was gently swaying in the breeze and the muscles were rippling across his body as he spoke. "Who is really to say that only humans can access consciousness? We are taking the human word for that, which we all know is limited by the data they put in their mind and the measuring tools they use. Is it not true that a vast number of poses and *pranayamas* in Yoga arose out of observing animals just like all of us? That unlike the Human, we already connect to and are guided by the Universe that lays within us? We can find water without Google maps, birds know when the weather is shifting, and turtles find their way back to their place of birth without GPS. I think what you meant to say is that we don't have that ego, the sense of I. But we are as creative, if not more, in how we choose to survive. But yes, the human mechanism is so sophisticated that if they could connect to their pure consciousness, the world they could create would truly be magnificent, for all of us."

Lion slowly lay down and bowed his head to Ocean. "I apologize for the interruption, Ocean. I feel we are becoming underrepresented on Earth, and I wanted to be heard by a human. Please go on. I shall refrain from roaring out my thoughts."

Ocean gently lapped at Lion's paws. "It is okay. You only spoke what we all feel. Now Corey, if you don't mind, I will explain consciousness to you as it is in Yoga, with AUM. I ask permission because I know when most humans hear that word, they think it is part of a religion, or a cult. It is neither."

Corey looked across Ocean at all the marine life that had arrived in the brief time he had been there. There were dolphins, turtles, whales of every type, sea birds, fish, and so many more for which he had no labels. It was extraordinary to experience animals from a place of no labels. He had no choice but to observe and feel them from a place of openness instead of limiting them to a predetermined set of boundaries often set around likes, dislikes, and emotions from the limited perspective of the human mind.

"Yes, please do so Ocean. I have taken off all my filters and hear you with an open heart and a quietened mind."

"Then let us begin but by no means end today. This will take more than one conversation. Also, please know that every part of the story of Yoga we tell you is just the tip of the iceberg. Humans have written entire books about each story, and there is a depth to each that is as deep as I am.

What we seek to do here is to make this story accessible to all humans and to give you the tools to engage in the discipline of Yoga, from the moment you begin to listen to what we are all about to share with you. This knowledge was meant to be shared. Only then will your entire species do what you were meant to do: Create and move forward the evolution of the entire planet in line with the visualization of the Universe.

There are four levels of consciousness, which are represented by the symbol of AUM and the little dot, the *bindu*, that sits separately from it, but is a part of it. AUM can be likened to myself, the Ocean.

The 'A' represents the conscious waking state, the one you are in now. It is the level at which humans experience the gross realm of existence."

"Sorry to interrupt, Ocean, but what do you mean by 'gross'?" asked Corey as he sat on a rock with his feet dangling in Ocean and speaking into the reflection of Moon. Whale had moved him there before she dove back into Ocean to replenish her energy.

"Gross elements are comprised of the five elements: earth, water, fire, wind, and space. In combination, they are in all the things you experience in the world external to yourselves. Gross is matter that is more tangible, like a rock, a tree, a river, etc.

Ocean Explains Consciousness

At the level of the thinking, waking conscious mind, your sense and action capacities take information from the outside world and enter it into the gates of the other levels of consciousness. Think of it as the surface of my body. As I move around the globe, I take all the information that is around me and absorb it into the layers below the surface. In your world, it is like a computer that takes in all the data that is external to it and moves it onto a hard drive where it is processed.

However, like you, I do not only take things in from the outside and process them within. There are also thoughts, driven by *samskaras* or ingrained habits, that rise from the bottom of my Ocean bed up to the surface that seek to be satisfied and acted upon by the mind. Don't worry, we will come to the mind in good time.

Just below this waking state, where all the thoughts and emotions swirl around your mind, is the dream-like state known to you as the unconscious mind and symbolized by the U in AUM. It is the huge body of water that exists below my surface. In this body sits the five main elements, water, air, earth, wind, and space, in their subtle energetic forms. Whereas the gross physical body is made up of bones, tissues, organs, nerves, etc., the subtle body is represented by *prana*, the vital energetic force in its totality; koshas, the layers of the energetic bodies also known as sheaths; *nadis*, through which energy moves in you; *chakras*, the places where many *nadis* intersect; and the *vayus*, the vital energetic winds that drive essential functions in your body that process and put energy to use.

Although the subtle bodies exist in your unconscious mind, they experience the world through your conscious waking mind.

Then there is the subconscious mind, which you can liken to the bed of my Oceanic body. Humans know it as the deep sleep state, and one I hope I have not put you into, Corey?"

Corey laughed. He now sat on the back of a turtle, large enough to sit three of him. The lives that lived in Ocean were gently passing Corey among themselves, each wanting to touch and feel the Human and to hear his energy, his Soul (soul), instead of his mind that constantly sought to dominate their world rather than allow them to just be.

"No, not all. Instead, I find myself wanting to stay here forever and learn. I am beginning to understand that what we humans call 'intelligence,' is very different from knowledge and, in fact, holds little worth in the greater scheme of existence."

"You have done well, Eagle, to bring us such an open human. And yes, Eagle, a handsome one as well," laughed Baobab, shaking all the animals that covered every inch of her limbs.

"Let us finish. Soon the sun will take my place, and Corey will have to return to his species. The 'M' in AUM represents the subconscious mind. It is where everything that has ever been input into your mind rests, where your thoughts, impressions, *samskaras*, known to you as your deep-seated habits and addictions, sit. Let's put it another way, shall we? In this deep sleep state, all the impressions you have absorbed from birth and even in former incarnations lay in their latent form. It is where the roots of your *samskaras* (habit patterns) and the driving force behind *karma* (your actions) are grounded.

Those wants, wishes, attractions, aversions, and desires that play out in your unconscious dream state that often transform into actions, speech, and behaviours in the external world via your conscious waking state all have their roots in the subconscious. Think of each impression as a seed at the bed of my Ocean. When watered with attention and energy, they begin to grow into trees that breakthrough into the unconscious and eventually into the conscious mind. Here, they emerge as full-blown adult trees that refuse to leave. Trees that then influence your thoughts and behaviours. And the only way you can cut down that tree is by burning the roots and the seeds that sit in the subconscious.

Thoughts and impressions from the subconscious emerge in two stages. The first is in the potential form, where they lay dormant before rising to the surface and being converted into action. The second are those that have already manifested into action. It is much easier to control and neutralise the latter than the former. We will go into what it means to control and neutralise an impression further on in the story. For now, understand that when you meditate, you can bring latent impressions to the surface and observe them. Once observed, you can decide what to do with the impression and even trace it back to its origins.

By accessing the subconscious through the process of meditation, you can access *samskaras*, the ingrained habits from mental or physical repetition, in their latent form. You can also observe all the impressions and habits that control your actions, your desires, behaviours, etc. It is here that you begin to understand that you are, in fact, being controlled by your thoughts and impressions instead of the other way around.

It is through your human form that consciousness seeks to evolve, to let go of the ego and purify the subconscious of its bondage to all *samskaras* and impressions such that it may connect to the universal consciousness. Contrary to popular human belief, your consciousness (soul) has not entered the human form to evolve the body that you humans seem to be so preoccupied with.

The whole human journey is one of involution. To begin to un-attach from the gross, the physical, and move back inwards to the Soul. Doing so liberates the soul from its entanglement with the natural human form, a form that you humans so strongly attach to that it creates mass suffering because it is by its very essence impermanent. Because your form is part of nature.

And remember nature is made of *gunas* and elements that are constantly shifting, changing, and seeking balance. Once liberated from your attachment to your form, you are free to use it to experience this limited life you have been given, without suffering. In this liberated state, which is *samadhi* (enlightenment), you can not only harness the power of your nature, but of all nature. So yes, those superheroes like Dr. Strange were not kidding. Those powers exist in all of you.

But this last state is one at which few humans arrive. Do not panic because without ever reaching that state, the human can still achieve a life of unending peace and joy and the power to influence their destiny.

Is it not funny, Corey, that it is in this deep sleep state, where you humans believe very little goes on, that the supreme knowledge, *prajna* resides? The place where you may begin to access what we in nature know to be the infinite library of wisdom and the root of the three *gunas*, the forces on matter. For it is there that they are constantly mixing in different combinations to influence the subtle elements in the unconsciousness, which, in turn, move the gross elements in the conscious mind."

Corey looked across the Ocean in awe. "Eagle," he whispered, "how is it that we humans don´t know any of this? Why is it not taught in our schools and our education systems? I know we are just at the tip of the iceberg, but I am already beginning to understand myself a little better."

At that moment, I wanted to wrap my wings around him, fly him up to Sky, and then to the bottom of Ocean, but I knew now was not the time. Ocean had one more layer to reveal before it was time for me to say goodbye to the Human again.

"Now, allow me to conclude here. Below all those layers of consciousness sits your Soul. It is symbolized by the little dot, or *bindu*, that permeates the silence after the vibrational AUM that humans chant. You can liken it to the earth that lies below my seabed. Separate from it but connected to it because it gives rise to the Ocean above it.

Ocean Explains Consciousness

When you reach this connection to your soul, it is called *samadhi*. From this viewpoint, you are not only able to witness all the layers of consciousness, but also influence it. But more importantly, in this fourth state, you begin to understand that the self, the Soul, is not separate from but collectively part of the absolute reality that pervades everything. I believe in your world of religions you refer to that collectiveness as God, whereas we call it the Universe."

At this point Moon let out an enormous yawn that nudged all of nature out of its meditative state and back into waking consciousness. "Corey," Moon smiled, "it is time for you to go back to your species. Who knows what will happen if they think you have gone missing?"

At this, Orangutan swung into the air, did a somersault, and landed on Earth just in time to give Corey a helping hand off Turtle's back. "I know. We would have a band of humans in layers of clothing running around here with guns and probably cages, trying to arrest us for capturing one of theirs. Their perception would be so limited that they would never believe Corey came voluntarily. Then, they would come back with all these machines, because they no longer believe in a fair fight, and try and clear us out to make sure that we don´t kidnap anymore humans."

Corey watched in amusement as all the animals rolled around in laughter. The flowers radiated more colour, the trees swayed, and Earth vibrated. He thought they were not far off the mark. "You are right. I should leave because until our entire species moves toward the light, you should fear us. Most of us do not see you at all. But before I take leave, please allow me to salute you. I have been practicing my moon salutation."

We all watched in amazement as Corey stood before us, raised his hands into the air in gratitude, and then proceeded to do a whole moon salutation. When he was done, he came back to mountain pose with his palms together, thumbs to his heart, head slightly bowed, and said the following words:

"May you all remain well until we meet again. May you know that I am grateful for all of you and understand that we are deeply connected and not separate from each other. May you always be a part of life, and may you know that every time we meet, the light in all of you begins to shine within me."

As he ended, we all bowed back to him and let out the most beautiful AUM I had ever heard. And in the silence that followed, we all disappeared into one vibration before slowly coming back to our forms.

"Eagle, will you fly me back to the place where we take our separate paths?" he asked shyly with his head still slightly bent.

"It would be my pleasure." And with no more need for words, we slowly ambled away from the place where magic was beginning to grow out of the seed we were all planting into the human's subconscious.

We moved in silence, each enjoying the aura of the other. It was a wonder to feel how in just a few short dates, yes, I was totally calling them dates, he had already begun to quiet the mind. I could feel a love rise in me that I had not felt for another species. It felt warm and comforting.

"Thank you," he said as we reached the fork in our path. "I try not to think about how all this has come about because I would drive myself crazy doing so. All I know is that it feels right and it was meant to be. Although I must tell you that when I walk back into my world, my mind tells me that I am not worthy of all the love you give me. That at some point you too will vanish once you really see me. You do know, as a human, I have more boxes than a game of tic-tac-toe. When I have sought love in the past, I believed that the only way I would find it was if the other filled all my boxes: religion, lived near me, looked and dressed a certain way, had a job that suited me, and so forth. But I feel love for you, and I think it is safe to say you fit not one of the boxes I have put love into, the main one being human." At this he laughed heartily. and his whole being quivered.

"If I told people at work that I was falling in love with an Eagle that I don´t feel worthy off, they, for sure, would have my head checked."

I could not help but smile and spread my wings. "Ahh, Corey, what you do not know is that I already see you. I see all that sits within you, and it does not scare me or make we want to fly away. Your fears, thoughts, your likes, your dislikes, they are not you. They are your mind and all that you have allowed to enter it. Then once planted, you have watered it with attention for years and years by attaching who you are to those thoughts and impressions. Give us your time, and, in return, we will show you who you really are.

But more than that, we will teach you how to change your thought forms because thoughts are how you interact with life and love. And every thought is energy, and all energy contains consciousness, as you now know. You can now see that thoughts are some of the most influential of all energies in the cosmos. When you have learnt to control your thoughts through meditation, contemplation, and prayer, well, then, Corey, you can create change in you at the most profound level, but more importantly in the consciousness of the collective."

With that, I landed on his shoulder and rubbed my head along his back, such was my balance and flexibility. For a moment, I lay my head against his heartbeat, and then I rose to the sky, bidding him farewell. For a moment, I watched him look awed by the glow of love that surrounded me, and then I flew back to that place where I was seen.

5

The Elephant & the Human Mind

As I arrived at the place of magic, I was forced to land on the back of a dolphin. It seemed the earth had transformed into webs, wings, hoofs, paws, feet, fur, manes, trunks, and a variety of shapes and forms the likes of which I had never witnessed. Instead of one Baobab, there were now trees of every kind housing animals from around the planet.

"There you are, Eagle. I had to call in for reinforcements for my branches were about to snap in half. It would seem that there are very few corners of the world where humans have not invaded us. Their lack of self-awareness and desire to survive at a level that is most obviously unsustainable is killing the rest of us. They seem to believe that to survive and find happiness, they need two cars, two TVs, two mobiles, closets of clothes, racks of shoes, three massive meals a day, marble countertops, fridges that speak to them, and lights everywhere. Something's got to go for them to have all that, and that something is us.

The story we are telling here through our thoughts and in the vibrations of our words has spread across the planet. And, as you can see for yourself, everybody wants to understand the human. The hope is that understanding may ensure their own survival."

"Dear Giraffe, do you mind if I just perch on your head for a moment such that I may address nature?" I asked the giraffe standing closest to me.

"Not at all, Eagle. Stay as long as you want. I have missed this connection to different energies and how they serve to lift mine to a higher level. Especially as all I feel is love around here."

I lifted my wings, flew onto elegant Giraffe's head, faced the cacophony of magnificent colours that pleased my vision, and then whistled. The quiet spread like a wave as everyone settled

The Elephant & the Human Mind

into their places after having spent the last hour establishing energetic connections. There was no jealousy, competition, insecurity, dislikes, or likes that plagued us as they did the human species. No, every being that was here had eaten, slept, or procreated before they arrived and therefore engaged in what was left over: love.

I would use telepathy. That is how we spoke with each other when the human was absent.

"Namaste beings. Thank you for coming to this place of magic. I ask that you remember that the Human carries a soul that is connected with all of ours through the hub of the united consciousness known as the Universe. Unlike us, the human mind sits in one of five states, and most often in the first three. I explain this to you today, so you can engage with humans from a place of kindness and understanding of just how deeply they are under the influence of their mind.

The first state is *kshipta*, which means a state of agitation and complete distraction. It is the lowest state, and here the mind is overly active, restless, and wanders like a nomad from one place to another. It is famously known as the 'monkey mind,' and it is where most humans live their waking lives. The monkey mind is dominated by the *rajasic guna*, which always seeks to be doing something: watching TV, scrolling on the phone, listening to music, browsing on social media, working, exercising, and so forth. In this state, a human is at the mercy of their thoughts and emotions with a complete lack of awareness of their behaviours. For these humans, meditation is a battle and access to self-awareness an impossibility.

Then there is the second state, *mudha*. The dull, lethargic mind, which feels as heavy as a bowling ball and very forgetful, a little like a donkey. Here, the human is lazy, unproductive, and seeks to zone out as often as possible. Although more settled than the first state, it still allows the mind to control a human rather than the other way around. Many humans also live in this state.

Third, there is the *vikshipta* mind, which so often disturbs the human attempting to meditate. I have heard this state called the 'butterfly mind.' It is not as bad as the first state because a butterfly can be cajoled for a moment to be still and focused. But even here, it is easily distracted by some attraction or aversion to something that then causes it to flutter away. Here, the *sattva guna*, the *guna* of calmness, begins to move into dominance. In this state, a human mind can easily be trained, and it is this state that I believe our human Corey's mind sits in.

With time, we will collectively move his mind to the state of *ekagra*, or one-pointedness, where the state of meditation is possible and the practice of Yoga begins. We like to think of this as the Eagle mind, where the human will no longer be distracted by internal or external activities and will comfortably rest in the awareness of the present moment rather than in the past or anticipated future. In this state, thoughts are uncoloured and moved back to neutrality, the karmic bonds of *samskaras* (habits) are loosened, and the human can enter the last state, *nirodha*.

Nirodha is where the movement of the mind field and all its inherent thoughts and emotions are ceased and quietened, where humans can dis-identify with the mind and remain as pure consciousness. It is like the earth below the oceanic mind, from which all rises but which is not identified or attached with that which arises from it.

In the present world, humans' experience of their reality rises from their mind, from the mental. Mind is an agent of *prakriti* and therefore of nature. It is one of the most subtle parts of it. So be kind to humans. They are enslaved by their mind and know nothing different. Their soul has been covered with more layers of ignorance than the largest onion on the planet. We are lucky that we have this human to speak with. He is open and seeks change and his true purpose. But just as important, he is deeply religious and part of the largest growing church in part of the human world. His journey with us will show all humans that Yoga offends no one and can be embraced by all of humanity.

Who does not want to live a life from a place of enlightened joy and peace?"

Just then, a flock of parrots that looked like a rainbow flying across Sky called out the arrival of the Human. I bowed to nature and then launched off Giraffe's head, expressing my gratitude for his patience and steadiness, then flew toward the Human. My heart was beating so loud that I was sure he could hear me before he saw me.

As I approached him, I saw him lift his head. A smile burst forth as he waved to me. I landed gently on his shoulder and stuttered in nervousness.

"Hello Corey, how wonderful it is to connect with you again."

He reached up, stroked my wings, and blushed slightly as he did. "It is nice to see you, Eagle. You have haunted my dreams."

I laughed so loud that I fell off his shoulder and landed in front of him. He stopped abruptly before he fell on top of me, although that might not have been such a bad thing.

"I hope in a good way. Do I still come to you as an Eagle? Or have you moved past the physical and into my formless soul?"

"No, still the physical, which is why I said haunted," he said still blushing. He was beginning to look like a rose with two arms, two legs, and solid muscle.

"Let's not touch that one, shall we? Come, let's go. The orchestra of nature awaits you, and Sun would like to greet you before it takes leave."

We ambled along in silence as I gently moved him into the present. With each step, he shed his roles as lawman, religious man, father, jitsu teacher. Thus, when he stepped into the cove, he arrived as just Corey. I knew as we rounded the bend and dropped into the cove that it would take him a moment to adjust to the forest that had arrived over the weeks and all the beings from across the world.

Yoga, Where the Impossible Meets the Possible

He was so absorbed in me that he did not hear all the chattering. As he rounded the bend, the chattering stopped, and his mouth fell open. His feet got stuck in shock. Mouth still open, he turned to me, speechless. I have to say, I kind of liked him in that state.

"Yes, Corey. Yoga is magic. Once the planet looked like this, when we were the majority and life was present everywhere in all its energetic forms. There was diversity of form and colour everywhere, and humans were once apart of that as well. There were no concrete jungles, no trash floating around everywhere, no cars nor pollution. There was just this vibrancy."

"Hello, Corey!" bellowed Baobab. "It is nice of you to return. It is amazing, is it not? Take a moment and drop out of your mind and into your body. Just feel the change in your emotional state from your world and into ours, which really is your world as well."

For a moment, Corey closed his eyes and absorbed all the sounds, movements, and energy that hugged and held him. He felt the loosening of knots that had blocked his channels and made him feel heavy at work and in his life. He felt space opening in him and a lightness that had alluded him for much of the week. With each exhale, he felt fear, anxiety, and stress exiting his being. With each inhale, he felt lighter, cleaner, happier. Although he was a minority, he did not feel it. He felt a part of something much bigger than himself.

He slowly opened his eyes, bought his hands to his heart, and said, "Namaste my friends. Thank you for welcoming me back. I am deeply grateful."

With that, every living being in the massive cove began their salutations. Some moved through them, some sat in stillness, others stood on their head or on their shoulders, but by the end they all came to stillness. With their hands over their hearts, without needing to be cued, they all inhaled and began their AUM. It was an AUM filled with knowledge, an AUM that

The Elephant & the Human Mind

dropped all their differences and united them as one in the silence that rose from the sound. It was magnificent.

When they were done, the largest elephant I had ever seen sauntered over to Corey and lifted him with his trunk onto his back. I, of course, needed no such assistance.

"Hello, Corey," radiated Sun. "Today we move a little deeper into Yoga for today we will begin to explain the mind to you. By 'we,' I mean the elephant on whom you sit. Elephant here holds intelligence and an emotional depth from which any human would benefit, so we thought it only fitting that he tell you the story of the mind."

Corey could only nod as we challenged all that he had learnt to be true. He had believed for so long that reading papers, magazines, and textbooks and watching podcasts and YouTube increased his knowledge without understanding that all he was doing was adding layer upon layer of ignorance. True knowledge, they were showing him, could only be obtained by going within, by tuning into the self and then viewing all that was external to him from a place of knowledge and not ignorance.

Because every experience of suffering and joy came not from the experience but from the mind's interpretation of that experience. If the mind was filled with fear, negativity, hatred, and anxiety, then that is how the human would experience the world. The mind determines one's reality. But to understand all this, a human required knowledge of the self, and it was not a knowledge that could be acquired in schools or universities.

The deep rumbling voice of Elephant brought me out of my contemplation and back into the present.

"Let us begin, shall we? In the yogic tradition, the mind is not the brain. Instead, the mind is made up of four parts, or functions. In the Upanishads, one of the oldest texts known to humans, the mind is described as four spokes of a wheel. The never moving centre hub is the self, the Soul, around which the mind seems to rotate. When the human is connected to the self, it uses the mind to manifest itself as well as to purify the soul and bend nature to its will rather than the other way around. Only in a pure, controlled mind can the soul see itself in the clear reflection of the mind. When the human remains unconnected to their true self because the mind is foggy with illusions and coloured impressions, it operates almost independently of the self. The mind, Corey, is impressive. It can either be the entity that saves you or tries to kill you.

The first spoke of the mind is *chitta*, which at its simplest level is the unconscious storehouse of all impressions, *samskaras*, cognitions, perceptions, and memories. It can be likened to the subconscious and the pure unconscious layer, the bed of the ocean and the body of water above it. The M and the *bindu* in AUM. Some may go so far as to say that it is aided and abetted by the hippocampus in the brain, the hard drive that stores all that enters through the human senses, and the amygdala, which plays a pivotal role in tagging emotional experiences such that they may be remembered or triggered in the future. Unlike the brain, however, *chitta* permeates every cell in body, in every living being.

Chitta is the storehouse filled with everything that has been imported into you from birth as well as from your ancestors and your soul's former incarnations. Your soul, your pure individual consciousness, carries all the information and history from its journeys before it entered the human form. Upon entering the human form, it loses all memory of anything prior to its birth due to the sheer power and complexity of the form, which buries the soul.

That, my friend, is a whole lot of impressions. Luckily for most of you humans, these impressions rise slowly to the top and not all at once. If they were to rise all at once, you would go crazy, which I believe some of you have.

Chitta is forever moving; therefore, impressions are constantly rising out of *chitta* into the unconscious and from there into the conscious waking mind. These wave-like movements at the surface of the mind are called *vittris*. Sometimes these impressions are triggered by something external to you, and sometimes it is just the constant movement of *chitta* that give rise to them."

"You still with me, Corey?"

"Yes, I am, and it makes so much sense why I am constantly battling all the experiences that happened to me in my marriage even though the marriage disappeared a long time ago," Corey spoke with both awareness and sadness.

"Don't worry," I whispered to him, "in time you will understand how to detach and destroy those trees born of seeds that keep trying to strangle you."

As we spoke, Elephant walked over to Ocean and lay his trunk out. "Ocean, would you mind if I cooled my body down with some of your water?"

"Please, help yourself. My water is meant to sustain life but not to be taken advantage of or filled with trash."

"Ahh, much better," trumpeted Elephant as he slowly moved back into the trees. "Where was I? Ahh yes, the mind. Flying above the mind, which we have visualized as an ocean, are the *manas*, birds, that the impressions call upon to pick them up and satisfy them. They do this by taking them out into the external world or bringing something from the external into the internal. These birds take the thoughts and impressions and then use the ten senses to satisfy or fulfill them. These senses include smelling, seeing, touching, hearing, tasting, speaking, movement, grasping, eliminating, and procreating.

And these birds, the *manas*, are not guided by a thinking brain. You could almost say they are reactive. In addition to this, they sit in constant doubt, forever questioning and arguing without the ability to decide, judge, or discriminate. Should I do this? Should I not? These birds, the *manas* that carry out the fulfillment of desires, impressions, and thoughts, are not decisive.

Manas are made of a multitude of layers and are present across the entire body in every cell. Every cell in your human body has a phenomenal memory, just like ours," chuckled Elephant as he nearly rolled Corey off his back. "Not just of this life, but of the millions of years that your consciousness has roamed the Universe in various forms as well as from all your ancestors. In every cell, there is memory and intelligence, but not intellect. Intellect is reserved for *buddhi*, the third function of the mind.

Buddhi is the spoke whose job it is to make informed decisions. Think of it as the sky above oceanic mind. In the western human world, some would liken it to the frontal cortex, the thinking analytical part of the brain. It is the *buddhi* that a human must train to view what rises in the mind and decide clearly and logically what to do it. When the *buddhi* is clouded from being too tired or stressed, the *manas* will dominate and tend to follow the desire of the impression reactively and indecisively.

Now, the fourth function of the mind is *ahamkara*, known to you as the ego. But to understand the role of the ego, there is something you must first understand: the colouring of impressions. Please know that when I use the word impressions, I include all the other words you are familiar with: thoughts, desires, memories, *samskaras*, etc. In the ideal world, the yogic world, impressions are neutral, something to be observed that holds no power over your words, your behaviors, or your actions. In fact, what we seek to do in Yoga is to take all the colourings you have given impressions and return them back to neutral.

So, what does it mean to colour? Very simply, it is the taking of thoughts, impressions, and habits and then attaching an emotion to them. We will go deeper into this at our next meeting, but for

The Elephant & the Human Mind

now we must finish with the ego and send you back to your people."

"Ahem, Mr. Elephant," mumbled Corey in the most authoritative voice he could muster while sitting on an elephant who could squash him like a peanut. "Before you go on, would you mind if I sat under the tree for a moment? Your back is beautiful, but my human bottom was not built for such a skeletal structure, and my back is asking for some reprieve."

At this Earth shook, "You need Yoga *asanas*, Corey, to build resilience in your body. You should see some of the things we need to sit on for hours and hours. Some of us don't even have paddings, like many of you humans. Elephant, go ahead and bring Corey down and let him sit on me for a while and lean his back against Baobab."

Elephant chuckled as he gently lay Corey on the ground. Then he decided he too needed a rest, so he lay down beside him. If I did not know better, I would have said that Elephant was enjoying the proximity to a human without a gun or a camera. As he slowly lay his massive body down beside Corey, he lifted his trunk and lay it against Corey's leg. A lesser Eagle would have been jealous. I giggled to myself, imagining this is what a human would say. But alas, we loved without attachment. Corey was about to learn just how harmful attachment really was.

"Now where were we? Ah yes, the ego. Think of it as the wind that blows over the oceanic mind and attaches itself to all the thoughts and impressions that are arising from the memory bank that extends from the depths of the ocean that is your mind.

The ego attaches itself to these impressions that are rippling across the oceanic mind seeking satisfaction of some sort and then falsely identifies itself with them. For example, as it stands alone, an impression may have been coloured with an aversion or dislike, however, when the ego attaches to it, it attaches an "I" to it. So, now you have those famous human sayings "I like", "I dislike", or "I want". It is the I, the ego, that calls out to the *manas* which we have likened to birds, to satisfy or act on an impression that it, the ego, has attached to.

In some cases, the ego takes an impression that is neutral and, by attaching to it, takes ownership of it. It then colours the impression by attaching a past experience to it. The goal of the ego is not to create ownership of that which is not to be owned but to provide humans with a tool to make sense of events by making them personal and to help organize the self around the event.

Many of the impressions that arise in a human are habits. When they rise, if the *buddhi* is clouded by unawareness and ignorance, then the *manas* will manifest the habit through action. For example, you get up in the morning, and the ripple that rises to the top is the thought of drinking a coffee or smoking a cigarette. If the *buddhi* is tired or has already moved into the future or the past and therefore is not present to observe this rising thought, the ego will call on the birds to pick up the thought. They will then engage in the proper senses, leading you to partake in your morning habit of having a coffee or a smoke without you even really being conscious of it.

It is in this manner that we create habits so deeply grooved into the mind that they become *samskaras* like the grooves in a record. The record is the mind, and the grooves are the habits and thoughts that have been grooved into the mind through repetitive actions. Attach the ego to the groove, and you soon start to identify yourself with your habits and your thoughts. Then, before you know it, when asked who you are, your answers begin to sound like this, 'I am a smoker, I am a runner, I am a surfer, a lawman, a Mormon, I like diet Coke and ice cream.' Well, you get the drift.

Now, if you are present and your *buddhi* is functioning clearly, then you will ask yourself if you really need that coffee or smoke. You will be aware of what that habit is doing to you and

The Elephant & the Human Mind

will make a concerted effort to break a negative habit that is controlling you and limiting your life by keeping you living in the same roundabout circle of life dictated by habits (*samskaras*).

Then one day, the role, activity, or item that you have attached your ego to with the use of the word 'I' or 'my' disappears, leaves, or is lost. What happens then? Well, humans become lost and spiral into a place of not knowing who they are anymore.

This false identification with the ego to all the coloured impressions and data stored in the *chitta* (the ocean that is your mind), creates great suffering in humans because you believe yourselves to be your thoughts and emotions. This is a slippery slope. To attach to anything besides your pure consciousness, your soul, is to open the door to suffering because aside from the soul, everything, and I mean everything, is impermanent. Your body, your thoughts, your relationships, your job, your roles will all change at some point. Leaving a human in a constant state of flux and riding a roller coaster of emotions. I personally believe this is humans' Achille's heel.

And you do this because of your complete lack of knowledge of what the 'I' really is. In its true form, it is your pure consciousness, the soul, that sits below the ocean of your mind. It is a bright light that seeks to shine through all the layers and reconnect to the universal consciousness of which it is a part such that it may lead a life from the knowledge of the Universe rather than the insanity of all that is held in the mind.

The true **I** is needed to create the willpower to say, 'I can change my life; I can quieten the mind; I can see I am not my mind,' etc. But for most humans that **I** is lost in its attachment to the mind.

Now this may be okay for a while, if the impressions the ego is attaching to are positive, good, and kind. But alas, they tend not to be.

I see our time is up for today, Corey, so I shall end with a summary of all that I have spoken about today. All that sits in *chitta*, which permeates every cell in your body and stores all impressions, seek to be satisfied by the *manas*. This happens when they rise from the subconscious to the unconscious and into the waking conscious state. Here, they are acted upon by the *manas* through the ten senses and coloured by *ahamkara*, the ego. If the *buddhi* is active, then intellect kicks in and tries to discern the best action to take with an impression and/or thought, thus creating a response. If the human is lacking in rest, sleep, proper diet, poor exercise, and bathed in stress, thus clouding the *buddhi*, then the *manas* will create a reaction. This in turn will give rise to an ever-fluctuating false sense of self. You think you are just a collection of habits, other people's thoughts you have taken on as your own, illusions, and false truths because when not controlled, witnessed, and neutralized, the mind controls the human, not the other way around, and the true self remains buried."

"I believe it is time for us to end story time," Leopard said as he dropped from the tree to lay on the other side of the Human and causing me to fly up onto the tree.

"How are you, Human?" asked Leopard as he took out his tongue and gave Corey an enormous licking kiss that basically swallowed his face and left it dripping. "I am sorry. I have always wanted to do that, but, as you know, I would most likely get shot for kissing a human."

Corey wiped his face with his sleeve and grinning like a schoolboy who had just experienced his first kiss. "It's okay. It was actually better than a lot of kisses I have had. Yours came with no expectations or demands, so thank you, I think."

Corey slowly made his way to standing and looked up at me. He did not have to say it. I knew he was asking me to fly him back to his world. He placed the palms of his hands together, touching his heart, and slightly bowed his head. As he did, all of nature did the same. Elephant rose, and this is what he said to all of us, but mostly to the human:

"May you all be well. May you remember the source of your happiness lies within you. May you acknowledge that you are not your mind nor any of your organs. May you move through your life with awareness and break old habits by creating new ones that are based on love, kindness, and compassion. And may you remember to start every day from a place of self-love such that love may grow and spread to all living things and beings in the Universe." With that, he and every elephant in the cove raised their trunks and, on the exhale, released the most powerful AUM. It resonated through every cell that was gathered around us, and for a moment in the silence that followed the AUM, we all became one again.

I could see Corey's love well up in his eyes. As a tear gently rolled down his cheek, and he reluctantly turned to walk away. I could tell it was becoming harder and harder for him to leave. We began in silence, and when he was ready, I asked him if he was okay.

"It is okay, Corey; you can tell me anything. I know that your past relationship filled you with mistrust of love, the burden of feeling unworthy of love, and a fear of speaking your truth. It is hard to speak a truth if you don't know who you are and if you have defined yourself according to the thoughts and behaviours of others toward you. When you truly connect with the pure self within you, that fear will dissipate because you will be connected to love. No one and nothing will ever again be able to rob that from you as the love you hold for yourself will not allow it.

I know this may seem odd, but I have a feathered heart full of love for you. It is a pure love that asks for nothing but for you to receive it without fear. Yes, I too will fly away one day. These visits will stop, the world around you will change, the impermanence of all will continue, but the love that sits in our souls will remain. Because it is not a love from the mind or the body. These too are in a constant state of change. It is a love that arises from my Soul, and when the ego dissolves, that love will come from the universal consciousness where no dualities exist."

He walked on in silence, and I allowed him for I could hear him process my thoughts and feel their power. When we came to the place where duality emerged and we separated, he turned to me.

"Thank you. I know you understand that this is hard for my mind to process. My habits are as deep as they are wide and rule how I interact with life and love. I ask that you be patient with me. Only now am I beginning to see this is a long journey and one that takes effort and work. I want to take the path to awareness of my true self such that I too may love you from a place beyond our forms. I have never met anyone quite like you. You radiate light and love to all those that cross your path, and you have trusted me with this story of Yoga. I am deeply grateful."

"As am I."

He moved slowly toward me and then bent down and kissed the side of my beak. For a moment, I could hear nothing but the beating of my heart in my ears, could see nothing but light, and my physical form erupted into energy that sought to be liberated. When my sight returned, I could see him looking down at me with a smile that told me all I needed to know. Yoga had begun to work its magic.

There was no more need for conversation. We each turned toward our destination and waited for the next moon.

6

Human Suffering & the Stars

Every time I flew to the meeting place, I was amazed at the diversity of nature that continued to gather. You only had to look across the forest kissing Ocean to know that the creative source of the Universe was magnificent. Only something so great, so inspiring could give birth to all these living forms on the planet that included waterfalls, valleys, rivers, cliffs, and mountains. All of it, really. I was excited about today; we had asked Corey to come on a night when every available star in Sky and the Milky Way would show themselves to the human. It was they who would tell the story today, the story that would provide an understanding to the root of all suffering in humans.

But that joy dissipated at the speed of a lightning bolt as I arrived at the forest that met Ocean, tucked away in a large bay behind a formidable cliff. There was something amiss, and I could feel it. A great sadness made its way through me and buried all my other emotions. Normally there was chatter and laughter, but today there was silence and sadness that pervaded everything down to the tiny leaves that sprouted from the trees.

I landed on Baobab and began to listen to the story Lion was telling. He sat at the edge of Ocean facing Sun as Earth rose to set it with the forest on one side and Ocean on the other. Wind ran its current through his exotic mane as he bowed his head slightly, devoid of the energy he needed to hold it up. In the wind, we all tasted and smelled his pain.

"I came here and left my pride behind. I needed to understand the evil in the human, to find a way to make peace and understand their actions. I was hoping to learn that they were not inherently evil and birth hope that they might stop killing us.

Do they not know we have a soul as well? You only have to watch our young when they are born. The personalities in each are so diverse. Each bearing the same genes, born of the same parents, in the same plains of Africa, yet every cub is different, manifesting a different consciousness. We too are living souls on a journey that feel pain, joy, happiness, and suffering.

Last night, they arrived in a pickup truck full of humans with rifles and placed a leg of meat on a tree. Of course, we did not know that humans had done this as we do not hold such thoughts. The females in the pride just smelled meat. They were hungry. They had been for a while as the land we hunt on has become smaller and smaller. More of it has been taken up to feed the human population that seems to have no limits, just like their appetite.

Two in the pride went out searching for the source of the smell, one was pregnant with a cub of the pride. Our choice is always to hunt for our food; it is the way of our life. However, stress, hunting, poaching, lack of water is slowly killing us all off. In the beginnings of the humans, we respected them. They hunted on foot, and the fight was fair. They killed just to meet their needs and to survive as we all do. Then something changed, and we became a sport, a trophy, parts to be used to increase vitality and fight off death. And why? For reasons based on illusions, ignorance, and the ego.

When the females found the meat and climbed upon the tree, they shot both, ripped their skin off, threw the baby away, and left what they did not need on the earth. They did not eat them or use them to save a life, but instead they took their skins and heads to adorn their walls and floors."

I could feel his heart constrict and the pain sear through his cells and his soul. His systems began to shut down as his body moved into stress. We all felt his pain. Humans did not understand that they created stress in us that had the power to kill us, just as it did them.

"I don't understand the humans," continued Lion. They are always seeking to cheat death and prolong life as if they value life, but yet they hold no value of life. They kill their own. They kill us for pleasure, for money, for sex, for power. That is not valuing life. In fact, it is their complete lack of value for life that leads them to behave as they do.

Did you know?" he whispered to no one and to everyone, "they raise us in cages for the sole purpose of hunting us? Why? Because it makes them feel like men. It gives them power. It fills their ego. Do they not know we all, from Cow to Rhino to Tree, bleed, wilt, and wither just as they do? That we have a soul, a vibration? That we are alive just like them? Are there any among us whose death looks pretty, happy, vibrant? Do your leaves and flowers not lose their colour, your limbs their lustre? Do we not go grey and get old? Have you ever seen humans keep a house full of dying plants? Do they not understand that we too experience emotions, but in our own way?

Have they never seen elephants mourn their dead or how we lions play with our cubs? How monkeys groom each other with care? How we love, oh, how we love. But we also suffer. Do they think when a fish struggles at the end of a hook and fights for its life that it is not suffering. Do they think that when a dog whines in pain that they are not feeling? We may not attach who we are to our emotions as humans do, but we still feel them.

You humans," roared Lion out into the world, "have removed yourself from nature as if you are somehow above it. You've become lazy in your desire for food and shelter and wanting it to arrive without hunting for it or building it. You have even wanted your companion to arrive over an app rather than going out to court one. In doing so, you have disabled the part of you that gave you purpose, meaning, and connection to the world in which you lived. But that yearning to create, kill, hunt, and gather remains in you. So, what do you do? You kill each other, hunt us for pleasure, and enslave yourself to money to meet your survival needs. And in so doing, you have lost your connection to all of nature and your purpose. You have lost the value of your food as you no longer have to work in the field or hunt, making it easier for you to eat excessively. As you no longer must build your homes, chop wood etc., you keep cutting us away to build bigger and bigger homes. You have lost the value of life as you are no longer connected to it.

I did not want to be the one to tell you this, but when you lost your connection to all of us, many of you moved from being survivalists that lived in balance with your surroundings to unknowing murderers. And how easy it has been for you to kill us every day in your ignorant yet convenient illusion that we have no soul or that you are not connected to us. Money and technology have given you the freedom to disconnect from life and from the consequences of your behaviours. Which is why you kill every day and feel no remorse at all. How often do you thank your food, the water you drink, the air you breathe, the earth you walk on?

Would you be so quick to kill if you had to chop the wood for your chair? If you had to hunt us on foot with a spear? If you had to harvest the field for your food? If you had to court and work for every act of procreation, as we do in nature? Would you kill us if you stopped blocking us out and heard us?

Believe it when I say that your peace, sanity, and joy lies not in ignoring us but in connecting with us. It lies in sitting with us and listening rather than describing."

We allowed Lion the space to move through his suffering, each of us sending him love and light. As we all sat in silence, none of us had seen Corey enter the cove. That is, until we saw him go down on his knees and place his hand on Lion's back. He bowed forward and laid his head beside his paw.

"I am so sorry for what we have done to you. I feel your suffering. Every day in my job I am confronted with the evil of humans, so that I too have asked myself over and over again if humans are evil beings. I have lived with these blinders like those put on horses for so long I cannot remember a time when I did not see humans as evil beings. Because of that, I have seen

Human Suffering & the Stars

the world in one way. I have limited what I have put into my mind to ideas and thoughts that support my beliefs. Therefore, my experience of the planet and its living beings has been filled with so much negativity and fear.

I am learning here that what I feed my mind, the filters and blinders I wear, become the sum total of my experiences and my life. It's like going to an amusement park and only ever riding the same ride because fear stops me from getting off my ride and onto one that is unfamiliar. As a result, my whole life looks like different versions of the same ride. The people, the speed, and the time change, but the ride remains the same.

I know you think we are evil, and until I met all of you, so did I. Please may you find it in your lion's heart to forgive us. We have lost our way because we do not understand ourselves or love ourselves. We are forever seeking our worth in such actions as killing, cheating, stealing, and relationships.

You know, a wise Eagle once told me that the best way I can protect you and change the world is by changing myself. She told me that when I struggle with change to remind myself to stay on the path of change not for myself, but for those I love because my change will radiate out in the world and touch all of those that I love like the ripples created by a stone thrown into a pond. Lion, by coming here I have stepped on the path of self-awareness and change not only for me, but also for you, all of you, as well as for my sons, my parents, and all those that I hold in my heart."

Lion slowly turned around and rubbed his mane across Corey's head. "Thank you. I needed to see the heart and kindness of the human and to be reminded of it. There are those among you who dedicate their entire lives to saving us from their own species. And, of course, I forgive your kind. The soul in me has taught me that besides gratitude, there is enormous power in forgiveness. Forgiveness is about freeing myself from the burden of suffering and you as well. To hold anger, resentment, and hatred is only to hurt myself. The seeds of such thoughts planted within me and watered, grow into trees, and I will see the world in this way. As a result, this is what the world will give back to me."

With that Lion raised himself on his hind legs and wrapped his front legs around Corey to give him the most enormous hug. In all my life as an Eagle, I never thought I would witness such an exchange of love and empathy between a human and an animal as large as a lion. The magic of Yoga never ceases to create surprise and wonder within me.

"Now, I think it's time for your lesson, and it is a lesson that I think will help both of us today," spoke Lion as he slowly raised his enormous body and stood beside Corey, who was dwarfed beside him. They smiled at each other, and together they walked toward Baobab after Corey took a moment to take in the growth of oceanic lives that had arrived. He was beginning to see how important this discipline was to the survival of the planet and all that lived on it. Well, more for those that lived on it because with or without us, the planet would survive and rejuvenate itself. It would be us who would disappear.

As he walked toward the tree, he looked up at me, and for a moment it was just us. I felt the warmth of his love wash over me, and in it I found freedom, not bondage and vulnerability as so many humans did.

"Hello, Corey. I speak for all of us when I say that it is nice to see you again."

"Thank you," he replied. "I am deeply grateful that I am able to be here." He placed his palms together, and we AUMed to reconnect all of us to each other and to the Universe within each one of us.

As the silence connected us to the collective energy, Sun disappeared, and what filled the void left behind was a sparkle that filled the entire sky. All the colours of the Universe reflected in the Milky Way. There were deep pinks that blended into soft purples, strong blues, and gentle oranges, each merging into the other such that you were not completely sure where one stopped and the other began. For a moment, every single being in every energetic form looked upward, mesmerized by the beauty the Universe had painted across the sky. We did not just see it; we felt the life within it and the promise of enlightenment.

The whole sky radiated love through our skin and into the very core of our souls, where it then slowly spread to every corner of our being: into our limbs, branches, petals, leaves, waves, and flippers. We could hear it sing a song so powerful and filled with so much light that it stole our breath away. Then it put it back into us and expanded it beyond our physical beings such that our breathing touched the sky and in the space between the exhale and inhale we all transformed into love and light. At that moment, we all knew that we were deeply loved, that when our forms disintegrated, our souls would merge back into the brilliance of the universal consciousness, this is what it would feel like. A love so strong that it could not be contained in our physical forms.

"Good evening," sang Sky. "It is wonderful to see all of you looking up instead of down."

At this, all the stars laughed, and the colours quivered. We could not help but laugh with them. "Human, we especially welcome you." The whole sky seemed to bend for the collective respect for this human was growing as they read his soul and felt his heart. In return, we all raised our arms, limbs, branches, waves, wings, flippers, and trunks to the sky and opened our hearts to what lay all around us.

"Beautiful!" came down the voice that seemed to come from everywhere above, from the stars, the colours, the blackness. "Now, I shall ask all of you to lay down on your backs. Yes, the trees and the plants as well. I know that flexibility lies within each of you. You are all yogis. What we are about to tell you is the root of all human suffering, and we do not want to add neck pain to that list."

For some minutes all that was heard was the sound of our forms as we all made our way onto Earth. As our bodies merged with Earth's and we felt its body envelop us into a hug and in our collective *savasana*, our heartbeats slowed, our muscles relaxed, and we became one with everything.

"Slowly spread your legs, your flippers, your wings, and your arms, so your palms are facing upwards. Move your shoulders away from your ears, toward which they always want to gravitate. Tuck your chin in toward your chest to align your spine and roll your shoulders in a little to protect your back. Human, if you have back pain, as so many of your kind do, you can also bend your knees, make your feet wide. and let your knees touch. Now just breathe, and with each exhale allow your body to sink into Earth and your heart to open to me, who lies above you."

And so it began:

"When you were last here, you learnt about the mind and all the impressions that lie, sit, and squat in it, coloured impressions that rise to the top of the oceanic mind and ripple outward. These colourings are called *kleshas*. Think of them as a collection of colouring pencils that colour all your stored impressions.

In the Yogic discipline, there are five types of colourings, or *kleshas*, that humans engage in with your impressions. For the most part, these coloured impressions create mental anguish and emotional suffering. From Sanskrit, *klesha* translates as obstacles, affliction, pain, and distress.

Now remember the bed of the oceanic mind, the *chitta*, where all your impressions sit. Well, some of those impressions are neutral and hold no power over you. They sit as a harmless memory. Some of them once had colouring, but through meditation, you have learnt to remove the colourings and bring them back to neutral by burning the seeds from which they rose. But, for many humans, your impressions remain coloured and give rise to tendencies toward action, satisfying *karmas*, or creating new *karmas*. More often than not, these colourings result in undesirable consequences and suffering.

Corey, remember that most impressions remain hidden in your subconscious. Rarely do they rise into your dream or waking state. However, when triggered, or due to the natural movement of *chitta*, some will rise into your consciousness waking state. It is only when they rise into this state that you are then able to witness the colouring of your impressions and the influence they have over your behaviours. These colourings distort your reality as they influence your perspective of the world around you, so often you end up perceiving a nontruth as a truth. Remember, Human, your reality, the way you see and interact with the world, is all in your mind. Think of the world and life as a large blank screen, perception as the projector, and your mind as the content reel.

The contents of your mind are constantly being influenced by five types of colouring. The first one, from which all the others rise, is known *avidya*, which translates into English as ignorance. *Avidya* is the foundation from which all the other colourings manifest at different levels. *Avidya* occurs when humans take a transient object to be everlasting, what is impure to be pure, and misery as happiness. It never ceases to amaze all of us up here that humans take stress, suffering, and misery as happiness. Tell me, Corey, how many humans do you know who would say they are happy? Many, right? Yet when you listen to them, you hear that they live in stress with their jobs, they have misery in their relationships, and they suffer in their transactions with the world. They have somehow mistaken misery for happiness.

In the Yogic discipline, what is meant by *avidya* is the deep-seated belief that what is not the self is the self. In other words, the ignorance of the profound truth that the only permanence in the Universe is the universal consciousness that resides in every living being as the soul, the true self. And yet humans continue to attach themselves and their belief in who they are to all that is impermanent because they believe that what is impermanent, transient, and ever-changing, such as the body, the mind, people, relationships, thoughts, emotions, and objects, are permanent."

"Are you understanding this, Corey?" asked the stars, the twinkle of which I could see reflected in his eyes.

Corey lay on the earth with Lion to one side, me on the other, Baobab at his feet, Ocean above his head, and ripples and ripples of nature around him. "Yes, thank you. I do. Please go on. I am excited to know the remaining roots that give rise to the suffering that seems to plague me."

"The second *klesha*, which rises from the first, is *asmita*, which translates as 'I-am-ness' or 'ego.' It is the sense of individuality that is created by identification with the mind/body complex. This is slightly different from *ahamkara*, the ego spoken of in relationship to the mind. This ego is the 'I' maker that takes that identification and extends it by attaching it to such things as gender, occupation, country, roles, etc.

In this *klesha*, humans create a false identity with the see-er, with that which it is seeing. Because of the ignorance of reality, namely *avidya*, the human associates itself with the limited body-mind complex, sense organs, sense perceptions, and intellect. This gives rise to this self-centred complex known to humans as the 'ego.' Because you attach who you are to these elements, you view yourself as a limited being. Additionally, you also see yourself as separate from the Universe in which you exist and which created you and resides within you, as well as from all other living beings of not only your own species but also other species. 'I am separate from the Universe. I am not a part of nature. I am separate from you,' and so forth. The human does not understand that all is one. They do not understand this because of *avidya*, ignorance of the true self.

Human Suffering & the Stars

In this state of 'I-ness,' you begin to have likes and dislikes, which takes us into the next two *kleshas*."

Just then, Sky exploded into a firework of shooting stars and a collective "ahhhh" rose from ground.

"You like, that don't you?" smiled the Milky Way. "It has made you feel all warm and magical inside, has it not?"

We all nodded at the same time creating a mirage of movement as the energy in all of us followed our physical forms.

"Now, the next time someone asks you if you like shooting stars, your human mind will dive into its memory bank to this experience, and you will most likely say, 'yes, I like shooting stars,' thus creating an impression of like in your subconscious to shooting stars and attaching that like to your identity.

This is the third *klesha*, *raga*, or attachment to your desires, the most dominant being happiness. When you see yourselves as 'I,' separate from all, you begin to be pulled toward objects, people, places, and things that give you pleasure. Let me try and explain this another way. Let's say, Human, that you meet a girl and when you are with her, she makes you feel happy and joyous. In time, you begin to attach your happiness to this person and believe that she is the source of your happiness. When this happens, you begin to fear losing that happiness, so you begin to cling to that person and move into insecurity, anxiety, and fear. But you don´t just do this with the girl. You do this with all things that provide you with a momentary, fleeting, or longer-term feeling of happiness. Then you add an 'I' to these likes, and voilà you have now attached your identity to that external person, place, object: my girlfriend, my car, my home, etc.

When you engage in this *klesha*, you hop on a merry-go-round of emotions. When desires of likes are fulfilled, you suffer because you fear losing that which you believe has created happiness in you. When you lose it, you suffer because you attached yourselves and your happiness to it. Only in connecting with your true self do you begin to understand that the source of constant contentment does not come from anything external to you but exists within you and in your oneness with everything.

The fourth *klesha* is the other side of the coin to *raga*, known as *devesha*, which translates into English as 'aversion.' This is the colouring of disliking things wrongly by avoiding things that make you unhappy. This is based on the false presumption that, once again, things external to you are creating pain and suffering in you. Human, let's say over time that girl you liked, you now dislike. Same girl, same reality, but now where there was once like, there is now dislike. She has not changed. What has changed is the colouring in your mind.

If she hurt you, you may even go a step further and attach pain to love, thereby colouring the tree of love with *devesha*. In doing so, your mind will now seek to avoid love because it has been coloured with feelings of unworthiness, jealousy, insecurity, and so forth because in humans, anything that threatens the 'I,' or the ego, is avoided.

This is sad, really, because just imagine how much of the world you are missing out on, how many infinite possibilities and opportunities you have closed yourself off to from liking and disliking things wrongly out of your misunderstanding that all these likes and dislikes are you rather than creations of your mind.

'I like this because it makes me feel good;' 'I don't like this because it makes me angry.' It is not the object that creates the like or dislike because then everyone that meets the object, person, place, or thing would have the same reaction. Remember the tire and how it is your mind that creates the colouring.

Now ponder on this: Just like the suffering attached to *raga*, most humans spend the other half of their lives suffering when they are unable to avoid a dislike or are subjected to a dislike.

Corey, when you re-enter your world, sit in awareness of how many of your actions and behaviours sit in one of these four following categories: seeking to get that which you desire, seeking to avoid that which you don't desire; suffering when you don't succeed in obtaining what you desire; or suffering when you fail to avoid that which you have an aversion to. For each of these states, there are a vast number of emotional reactions that include pain, jealousy, insecurity, and joy. In fact, nearly every emotional response that runs through you daily is in relation to one of these four scenarios. There are other reasons for emotions, but we will get into that later.

Before we move into the last *klesha*, why don't all of you take a little stretch?"

Corey slowly rolled to the side to protect his back. He then rose to a seated position and turned to me. I was grateful for the shadows that protected the change in my colour from laying beside the human.

"Yes, nature, rise and move your wonderful forms returning blood to all the areas that have been deprived of oxygen from the flow of blood pumped by your muscles."

In the shadows, it seemed as if Earth were rising then bending into a forward fold, stretching into a long dog, elongating its spine into a plank, and then releasing her back as she lay back down and lifted her chest off the ground. From here, Earth seemed to transform into a mountain as she moved into a down dog, then slowly moved forward to rise like the trees that were grounded into her, and then up to a standing position. Earth then seemed to fold back into a forward fold, into a squat, and then slowly back down to a place of feeling rejuvenated.

"And now we have arrived at our last *klesha*: *abhinivesha*, the fear of death based in the false belief that you are a limited being attached to your body/mind complex such that when it dies so shall you. For this reason, humans fear change because change leads to the loss of the things to which their identities are attached, the largest being the body. As a result, humans are constantly trying to control all that is beyond their control and transient with apps, medicine, stem cell replacements, chemotherapy, anti-aging tablets, Botox, etc. Alas, you are back to ignorance.

It is this constant fear of death that prevents so many humans from living life. Instead of living your lives, which is only ever the moment you are in, you are constantly seeking ways to preserve the life you are not living. As you believe that when you die, all of you is gone. That there is no immortal soul."

At this point, Sky and all her playmates took an enormous inhale and expanded themselves. On the exhale, their colours grew brighter, and we felt a warm breeze sweep over all of us.

"Corey, it is a result of all these *kleshas* that humans spend a vast amount of their lives in a reactive state to the world around them instead of a responsive state. You are always seeking to satisfy or avoid a desire from a place of ignorance."

I could feel Corey beginning to feel overwhelmed by the knowledge he had being given today, mostly because he did not know what to do with it. He felt as if he were being handed all the parts of an Ikea object without the instructional manual. I knew if I could feel it, then Sky could as well, so I waited.

"Now Human, I know the knowledge we have passed on today is enormous and can feel a little overwhelming, but be patient. As we move forward into the eight limbs of Yoga, we will hand you the tools to begin to un-colour your impressions as well as the tools to move through all the layers of the natural human form such that you may eventually connect to your pure consciousness.

On the path, teachers will enter your life to help you along. It is a path that requires guidance and teachers, depending on how far along the path you want to travel. But for now, know that what we seek to do here, in these magical meetings, is for you to begin to understand yourself and to give you the tools and guidance to gently move you off the path of suffering and onto the path of enlightenment.

Corey, I know you must wonder, 'what universal consciousness would create a form that endures so much suffering?' We will go more deeply into that as we move along, but for now please understand that suffering is important for humans. Only in suffering are the flames of desire to seek one's true self fanned. Only through suffering and pain is the soul purified.

When you suffer, you become aware of where you are stuck, aware of the actions and habits you keep repeating over and over again, and aware of the lessons that need to be learnt and the negative karmas that need to be broken. To do all this, you must first have awareness of all the above, and then, from there, shed your attachments to the human form and purify your mind.

Humans must seek out change that makes you feel uncomfortable, so you can clearly observe your mind. Observing your behaviours, reactions, responses, words, and thoughts toward people or events that challenge you. As you continue up the path of Yoga, uncomfortable situations and your reactions and responses to them will allow you to see how far you have involuted toward your soul. The more change does not phase you, does not create suffering in you, the less fear you have toward it, the more peacefully you move through it, indicates the closer you have moved to living your life from your Soul and not from your mind.

Now, please allow us to bid you good night and show our gratitude for your presence and openness today. This knowledge can only be conferred to those that are open to it as you are."

In the next moment, every single star and the Milky Way lit up, smiled down upon us, and collectively embraced us with their subtle electricity. An electric current moved through us sparking an awareness of our own vibrating energy. We all slowly rolled to our sides and up to a seated position. From there, we came onto all fours and rolled up vertebrae by vertebrae until we were upright again. We were alive.

I turned to Corey. "Thank you from all of us. We hope that you will return at the next full moon."

"I would love to never leave." He stared deep into my eyes, and I knew he meant not only this place with all its wonders, but also and more specifically me. "The minute I step into your world, there are no judgments, no fears, no insecurities. The layers fall away, and my Soul shines forth."

We all smiled at the subtle shift in his language, and then we AUMed to bring us all back into one with the Universe within each of us.

"Come, let me fly you back." We bid all of nature farewell and then sauntered back in the direction whence we had come.

"Wow. That was incredible," he sang as he smiled at me the smile that melted my heart every single time. Then he looked up at me, perched on this shoulder. "I missed you."

"I missed you as well."

"It is hard to stay present when you keep pulling my mind into the future," he confessed the thoughts that had sat in me as well.

"I understood today the impermanence of this relationship, but I also understood that if I can reach that connection to you with my soul, then we will be one forever." He blushed. I knew it had taken an enormous amount of effort for him to speak his truth without fear of it being rejected.

Then he continued, "It is my greatest hope that one day I will transcend into a form where I may experience all of you."

I laughed out loud. "In time, Human, all will happen as is meant to be. But first, I want to plant a seed in that handsome head of yours. As you move through your days, begin to be aware of your colourings and the influence they hold over how you interact with the world. Every human has a story, and thus every action that rises from them is a result of a conditioning and a colouring that has been implanted into them from the time they were born or, in some cases, well before that by their ancestors, or by karmas and *samskaras* from former incarnations. Have compassion for your enemy, Corey. They, like you, are a product of their mind. They too are broken, and they too have a soul that is connected to yours.

Seek to know their stories, so you may better understand them. The stories of those around you are important to help you understand their colourings and the basis of their ignorance. But it is also important for you to share your story, so others may understand the foundation of your actions and behaviours.

And in all this awareness of the source of your colourings, you will understand that there is never a need to engage in negative emotions, anger, annoyance, jealously, etc. You will understand that open and honest communication with yourself and with others will alleviate the need to engage in such emotions as you learn to live above them. Let me end with this: Humans are masters of creating stories in their heads, of believing they know what the other is thinking. This amazes all of us. Humans do not understand their own mind or brain, so how can they understand another's?

The basis of most conflict and suffering in your world rises from a place of misunderstanding and poor communication. Therefore, Corey, if ever you begin to create a story in your mind about me, please stop. Instead, the next time we meet, ask me and I will answer your questions from a place of self-awareness. Until then, ask yourself why you created that story, a story that is often one of suffering or of fantasy. What is it in you that choose the narrative you did?"

We had reached that place where our duality began to manifest, and here we paused for a moment as I let that seed sink to the bottom of his subconscious. I knew it was time for words to stop, so we spoke with our eyes and our energy. There was nothing left to say as what we really sought from the other was faith.

I gently rubbed my head against his as he lay his hand on my wings. I then lifted off him and into the sky before I gave myself a heart attack from being so close to him. I gently hovered for a moment and watched him walk away into the world that so strongly separated itself from the rest of us.

7

The Eagle & the Human Personality

I flapped my wings as hard as I could to that point of freedom, the place where I could just glide through the sky, swoop down cliffs, over Ocean's currents, and just be. I could sing as I moved through each present moment with complete and utter focus on that which lay in front of me while completely surrendering to the Universe that lay within me. I knew if I led from that vantage point, my life in this form would guide me so that it would be exactly as it was meant to be.

What all of us in the cove wanted humans to understand was this: Every human is predominantly a product of what they witness and experience from the time they are born. Therefore, it is no wonder the world looks like a washing machine stuck on the same cycle. The only way to break that cycle is to break the individual karmic cycles that humans are stuck in.

Every cell in the human body is pervaded not only by consciousness, but also by the memory of one's ancestors. From that one cell given to a human by each parent, 36 trillion cells spring forth, each holding decades of encoded memories of pain, suffering, bliss, and diseases of their ancestors.

These conversations with the human are so important to make all humans understand that if they do not want the lives of their children and grandchildren to mirror theirs, then they have to break their karmic cycle. That cycle can only be broken if they understand themselves, their ancestors, and why their consciousness chose the body and life it had.

Karma is one of the most misunderstood words in the human vocabulary. It can mean either 'action' or 'the result of action,' but it is mostly used to denote reactions to past actions. No action goes without a reaction, even if that reaction does not arrive until years later. When the time is right, a karmic reaction will rise to the surface and express itself. What causes an act in the first place are *khleshas*, the colouring of impressions, because neutral impressions hold no power and do not manifest into action or words.

When you do *karma,* you reap *karma.*

Yoga understands that it takes only one strong *karma*, a repetitive act, to give rise to the specific body and life into which all living beings are born because it is through a chosen form and life that karma can fully express its reaction. For example, if in a former incarnation you sat in a place of power and used that power to force thousands to change religions and punished them if they did not, then, at some point, that *karma* now inscribed in your consciousness will enter a specific body and life to reap the consequences of those actions. A life in which you may be beautiful and courted by powerful religious men, who will then abandon you because you do not follow their religion. Those men will not only arrive in your life for you to pay your karmic debt, but also to give you an opportunity to break that *karma* by learning to forgive yourself and to walk away from those men without anger or resentment.

Connected to that one strong *karma* that determines the next incarnation of your conscious energy, there are several smaller *karmas* that will likewise use the form to express themselves. Some *karmas* will be good, and you will enjoy the reactions to previous good acts. Others will be painful as *karma* is paying a debt. And all the while these *karmas* from pre-existing acts are coming to fruition, you are creating new *karmas* in this incarnation to be fulfilled in the present form or in future incarnations. No matter how pure you may try to live your life, once a *karma* has started its journey, the momentum of seeking to fulfill the reaction to the action will continue for as long as the body that the *karma* has allotted to itself remains. Although one has no control over past *karmas* and the reactions they will reap, humans do have control over how they will respond to those *karmas*, and in the creation of new ones. This is where

The Eagle & the Human Personality

Yoga creates lasting and fundamental change. It provides the understanding that a happy or unhappy life is one's own creation from one's own behaviours, thoughts, and actions.

I was looking forward to today's story because today we would begin to hand Corey the tools of change. My ponderings ceased as I began to approach the cove of magic. I knew Corey would already be there. I had asked Hawk to fetch him because I had been forced to travel a little further than normal to catch my food. Ocean was being raped by the humans' bottomless appetite for fish. I sometimes wondered if the problem was that there were just too many humans. Could you imagine what destruction eight billion elephants would cause to the planet? Is it not because it disrupts the whole ecosystem that humans cull us when our numbers grow too large?

I began to move into the present as I saw Baobab in my bird's eye. I could hear the chatter filled with joy rising off Ocean and Earth. It felt good to be back among all of them. As I landed on Elephant's back, a hush descended, and I could feel Corey's gaze piercing my soul. I knew the Human, so I knew he was wondering if he had done something wrong or if my love for him was as feeble as he had experienced love to be.

"Hello, my fellow beings. Thank you for waiting for me today. I am sorry I am late, and Corey I deeply apologise for not being able to escort you here today. No doubt Hawk kept you adequately entertained and was nothing short of charm. It is getting harder for us to find fish in the places where we once hunted. As we have, rightly so, put a moratorium on any of us in this magical kingdom eating the other, I had to travel further than normal to feed myself today."

Corey's relief was as tangible as was the empathy from all those who were gathered; most of them were in the same predicament.

"Now, if you don´t mind, I am going to take a little wash in the majestic energetic healing powers of Ocean. I shall cuddle a few of you that have gathered in Ocean and then we shall begin today's class."

I then flew back to Baobab and perched beside Corey. He had made his way to higher limbs, where he now sat surrounded by hummingbirds, bees, butterflies, ants, and caterpillars.

I began: "The spiritual journey, Corey, is not out in space, nor at a retreat, in India, at Mecca, nor in any app, nor in time. It is within each and every human. It is the path from ignorance about who or what you are to knowledge of your true self. And this, my human friend, is a mission because spirituality has been placed in so many boxes, such as religion, hippies, and hocus pocus, that humans shy away from it. You see it as brain washing, and rightly so, because knowledge has too often been misused by your species for power and money. Why is Yoga not taught to every human? Because this knowledge of the true self, if every human were to learn it, would dramatically change the world as you now know it. The world would shift from a place of fear that keeps being fed to humans in all media to a place of light, love, kindness, and compassion to all living beings and to oneself, thereby removing the influence of those in power over all of us.

How do you find that infinite conscious reality within? Fear not, we are getting there. First, you must understand where it resides in you. And thus, we have arrived at the *koshas*, the five interlocking sheaths of the human personality.

It is your attachment to all these sheaths that prevents you from knowing your true self, a self that pervades all the sheaths but is also separate from all of them. I will briefly explain all five of them to you today, and when I am done, we will launch into the eight limbs of Yoga, which I like to call the 'tool kit' to inner peace and happiness.

I know I said we would start the limbs today, but it may not happen. Sometimes even I forget the enormity of this discipline. Too often Yoga teachers and students reduce Yoga to half-naked photos of themselves in all sorts of contortions. Imagine if Buddhism were represented that way as half-naked teachers in meditative positions!"

I rolled my eyes and nature let out a chuckle, imagining what the Dalai Lama would think.

"Now Corey, follow me and I shall guide you through the layers or sheaths known popularly as your personality." By now the whole of nature had read my thoughts, and it was useless trying to hide my enormous crush, from a place of nonattachment, on the Human.

"Please know that the layers are not distinguished by their placement in the body but by how subtle they are. We will start with the layer that is most gross and slowly move down to the layers that are more subtle.

When asked, 'who are you?' most humans will point to their body, and say, 'this is who I am.' But is it really you?

The outer most sheath, the body as you call it, is known as the *annamaya kosha*, the food body. In humans, the entire skeleto-muscular framework, your organs, autonomous nervous systems, sense organs, and so forth falls within this sheath. It is a modification of what you eat and drink influenced by your lifestyle. I once heard someone say that the body is food rearranged. For this reason, it is also known as the earth body and the gross body.

But how can you be the body when the body is constantly changing, and yet there are so many aspects of you that remain the same? The body is an object that can be touched, felt, smelled, and experienced by the five senses, so how can you know the body and experience it if you are your body? You cannot. It is not possible to be both the knower and the known. When you look at the hand, it is you, the knower, observing the hand. It is not the hand observing you because how bizarre would that be?

Yoga, Where the Impossible Meets the Possible

When you begin to understand this, you stop attaching your sense of self to your body. In humans, this attachment to the body is what ages you. As the body begins to wither away, you age with it due to the attachment to your sense of self to it. Another way to view your body is to see it as the temple that houses your Soul. Therefore, it should be kept healthy because it houses you and because an unhealthy body will negatively affect all the other sheaths.

Corey, every philosophy in your world will tell you that you are not your body. Remember that you chose this body to satisfy your *karmas*. This body you hold is a tool for consciousness to experience nature and to purify itself. Your soul will continue to exist long after your body dies. If you are lucky and do the work in your next incarnation, you may just end up with the body of an Eagle."

At this, I smiled at Corey, and all of nature erupted, mummering on about "why not their bodies?" They all began to examine their bodies, pointing out the magnificence in their flippers, their colours, their trucks, and their flowers. I allowed the detour because it is always nice to acknowledge one's vessel and all its beauty from a place of non-attached observation. Though these days, humans were creating a definition of beauty through the media that was nearly impossible for anyone to attain and left most humans feeling just a little ugly. How ridiculous! Beauty radiates from the inside out, not the other way around.

That deep laugh we all loved so much moved from the belly of Earth upward and outward, vibrating us all into silence. "You funny beings, all of you. She said Eagle's body, because, well, you know why."

"Ahhhhhhhhhhhhh, yes," the chorus hummed in perfect unison, creating a transformation in the colour of Corey's body from luminous to red.

"Um, shall we continue?" I laughed, enjoying Corey's discomfort as in it his feelings were reflected outward instead of buried inward.

"Now Corey, each limb of Yoga contributes to the overall balancing of the entire body and prepares it for you to connect to your true self and not constantly be pulled by all the layers that come with being a human. Some limbs have a greater effect on a certain sheath than others. In the *annamaya kosha,* the greatest influencer besides a healthy diet and lifestyle are *asanas,* which in time we will dive into deeper.

So, now that you understand you are not your body and that you must be something infinitely more subtle, let's look a little deeper and see if we can find you.

The next sheath is the *pranayama kosha,* the energy body which is influenced by the health of the *annamaya kosha.* It is the layer associated with the movement of energy, the life force, through *nadis,* which Western science calls nerves and Chinese medicine calls meridians.

The movement of energy in your body is essential to maintaining the processes of digestion, oxygenation, and respiration. The flow of energy influences the processing, creation, and movement of chemicals and hormones. It also maintains the flow of blood that keeps your body alive, and so forth. All these systems are fueled through the use of breath to influence the movement of energy (*prana*) throughout your body.

This layer has more influence on your health than the gross body because it drives all your systems. In Chinese medicine, it is known as *chi,* in Yoga as *prana.* In both Chinese medicine and Ayurvedic medicine, it is this layer that they work on to bring balance and health back into the human, not the gross body layer that Western medicine investigates for health.

But like the first layer, this layer is also ever changing as *prana* moves like waves through the body. Sometimes you feel energetic, other times not so much. But you are still the same person, are you not? When you meditate with the breath, who is observing that breath? You are, so once again you are the observer, the knower, and *prana* is the known. You are conscious of it. For all these reasons and so many more, you are not your *prana*, you are something subtler. And like the first layer, it is important to keep *prana* flowing freely, without blockages and stagnation, such that you may go deeper into yourself.

The next layer defined in its simplest form is *manomaya kosha* which translates as 'the mental body,' or 'the mind,' and refers to your thoughts, your emotions, your entire personality. Most humans define themselves by their thoughts, feelings, emotions, likes, dislikes, and so forth. They say this is their personality. But hold on, are you not aware of your mind? Is the mind not something you experience? Is your personality not something you experience? Therefore, how can you be your mind? The mind is an object of knowledge, and you are the knower.

I once heard that humans have, on average, sixteen thousand thoughts a day. The vast majority are repetitive thoughts, not unique creative thoughts, because that would make all of you geniuses. In addition to this avalanche of thoughts, there are also a host of desires that compete for your attention constantly. These are many and you are one, so how can you be your thoughts and your desires?

Corey, did you know that the word 'personality' stems from the Latin word 'person' that referred to the masks worn by performers to project different roles or disguise their identities on stage? That is what your mind does; it creates multiple personalities through its attachments, all of which serve to keep you from knowing you true identity: your soul.

And this is where the journey of meditation begins, the place where, in the silence between breaths, you begin to observe the mind and realize that you are not your mind.

So let's look a little deeper, shall we?

The fourth layer is the *vijanamaya kosha,* also known as the intellect, the *buddhi,* or the frontal thinking cortex. Yes, it is a part of the mind, but here a distinction in function is made. The intellect seeks to understand through analysis and introspection. Is this layer you, Corey? You may think so because it is here that we most often use the word 'I.'

But are you not aware of this process in you when you say such things as 'I am confused,' 'I don't understand,' or 'I understand'? Are you not aware when you engage your intellect that you are doing so? If so, then you cannot be your intellect either because it is still an object of awareness, even if it is much more subtle than the other layers. As with the other layers, this too changes constantly, and yet you always feel the same. Remember Corey, the self is the unchanging witness of the intellect, the bed below the oceanic mind. As you move deeper into the layers of meditation, you will come to realize this as well.

Let's go just a little deeper into the last layer, the *anandamaya kosha,* a place few humans reach or even know exists. It is here that the sages, saints, mystics, and gurus separate themselves from most humans. It is the state of deep sleep where there is no awareness of the body, no dreams, and even you are not aware you are in deep sleep because the mind and intellect have shut down. Yet still something remains such that upon waking you can say, 'I slept like a log.' If there were no awareness of the depth of your sleep, you would merely say 'I went to sleep, and then I woke up.'

It is here that you meet the *anandamaya kosha,* the place of deep untroubled rest, the sheath of bliss. In this state, one experiences feelings of joy, pure love for all the Universe, and illumination. It can be reached in the highest levels of meditation once all the other sheaths have been purified. Some say the path to this sheath is through selfless service to all living beings and surrendering to the Universe that exists within and *samadhi*, the state of intensely focused meditation.

It is the thinnest sheath and closest to Soul or pure consciousness that, although it pervades all five sheaths, is not any one of them. I can see this is a lot for you, Corey, so let me summarize these five sheaths for you in a way that makes it a little clearer.

Look at your hand, all the bones, tendons, ligaments, and muscles that make it up. That is your *annamaya kosha*. As you lift your hand, the energy that enables you to lift it is the *pranamaya kosha*. The thought you engaged in to lift your hand is the *manomaya kosha*. The feeling that I am lifting my hand, the action, and identification with it is the *vijnanamaya kosha*. The joy you feel in lifting your hand, because perhaps you injured it and have not been able to move it until now, rises from the *anandamaya kosha*. These, Corey, are the five layers of the human personality, ever-changing, constantly transforming, while your sense of you remains steady. So, where is your true self if not in these sheaths?

Well, let me tell you a famous little story told among Yogis that may create some clarification for you. One day, ten friends crossed a river that was flowing quickly and filled with obstacles. When they reached the other side, they stopped to count if they were all there. One of them asked the others to line up and began to count: One, two, three, four, five, six, seven, eight, nine. 'Oh my gosh!' he wailed, 'the tenth one of us has drowned,' and they all began to mourn.

Another among them asked the others to stop sobbing. 'It is not possible,' he said, 'that we have lost one of us.' He asked them all to line up again, and this time he counted: One, two, three, four, five, six, seven, eight, nine. 'Oh no, you are right! One of us has drowned.'

At this, they all dropped to the ground and began to sob. Just then, a yogi walked by and asked them, 'why are you all crying?' Well, one of them explained that there were ten of us, we all crossed the river, and one of us drowned. The yogi took a quick count and counted ten, so he asked, 'how do you know the tenth one drowned?'

'Well, because we counted, and there are only nine of us.'

The yogi calmed them down and reassured them that all ten of them were there. He lined them all up and asked one of them to count again. And so, he began: One, two, three, four, five, six, seven, eight, nine.

'See?' he moaned, 'there are only nine.'

The yogi grabbed his hand, turned it toward himself, and said, 'you are the tenth.'

But they were still not sure, so one of the other friends tried the same thing. Voilà! All ten appeared. Upon discovering that they were all there, they erupted into great laughter.

Once they had released their worry through laughter, the Yogi turned to all ten of them and said, "Do not worry, humans do the same thing in your life all the time. You keep missing the Soul because you are seeking an object outside of your true self, in your sheaths or in the external world. The tenth one is not out there in the world or in your layers. It is you, the one who is seeking, the observer of all.'

The entire field of Yogic knowledge can be divided into the known and the unknown. However, there is also the knower. If you think the Soul is something you can know, then you are mistaken. If you think it is something unknown to you, then you are still sitting in ignorance. The Soul is the knower. It is the subject, not the object of knowledge.

I think that is enough today, do you not?"

Yoga, Where the Impossible Meets the Possible

"Yaaaar," purred Leopard as he seemed to rise out of a mental coma. "Corey, you humans sure have it tough. It is no wonder you suffer so much, attached to all those constantly shifting and transient sheaths. I gotta say that I feel pretty grateful to be a leopard, no matter how hard humans are making life for me."

As the next moment arrived, all of nature sprung to life and began to dance with their bodies. They used their breath to move *prana* through them, so they could do back flips, somersaults, rolls, jumps, sways, anything that their body allowed for. Today's story had made them all grateful that they were not human because they were learning that to be human was no easy feat.

Just when we had all forgotten about the Human, Corey jumped off the limb on which he sat and started to salsa with Orangutan. As he twirled and dipped her, all of nature stopped, and their mouths, beaks, petals opened and stared at him.

"Hey, Human," shouted Walrus, all his blubber wobbling as he did. "What are you so happy about? Have you forgotten you are a human?"

Corey stopped and slowly made his way onto the rock where Walrus splayed herself. He had the largest smile for a guy to whom we had just shown the layer upon layer he would have to work through to reach his Soul.

"I am happy because, well, there is light in my tunnel. There is always light when one learns knowledge of oneself because then there is hope for change, for a life different from the one I sit in now. It helps that I have started practising *asanas* and *pranayama* daily, which lends to such feelings of calmness and joy. But mostly I am happy because the more I understand myself, the more joy I find in experiencing the human form from a place of awareness and non-attachment."

When he stopped talking, we all stared at him for a moment, dumbfounded by these words. Then the moment passed, and the birds began to whistle, the whales began to beat the drum of their bodies against Ocean, and soon the whole of nature was playing their tunes and dancing in joy for the Human. When we had exhausted ourselves, I turned to Corey. "Shall we?"

"We shall," he replied.

He turned to the gathering and AUMed. Then he placed his hands on his heart and bowed his head.

"May you all be well until we meet again. May you be treated with kindness and respect from my species. May we learn to see you and acknowledge that the light that shines in you shines in us as well. May you be free to live from your places of love and not from fear of us. And may I wake up everyday in a place of gratitude for all the love and light you have poured into me from the moment you entered my life."

Nature bowed back to him, and we slowly walked back toward duality.

"Thank you, Eagle, for not giving up on me. As you can see, we are not simple beings."

I landed gently on Corey's shoulder. "Truth be told, it has never been my choice to make. The Universe has pulled me to you. This is our path. And for as long as we may walk it, I shall revel in the joy it brings me, layers and all.

But, I should warn you now, Corey, the more you follow this path, the more solitary it will become. As you change, fewer and fewer people will understand you, even though you will understand them because you were once them. But in that void, a bliss will rise that will accompany you everywhere such that loneliness is something you will never feel. Did you know that when you feel lonely, it is not another but yourself and your connection to your soul and to all of life that you are missing? Understand that you are complete just as you are, that when you finally connect, that loneliness will disappear and what will arrive in its place is solitude, joy, and a deep sense of peace with yourself.

This is why so many relationships fail: because humans enter them expecting the other to complete them. That is an impossible expectation to put on another, and on yourself.

Now I must leave you here." I rubbed my cheek against his. His smell, his energy, the feel of him, was beyond anything I had ever experienced. If only love felt like this for everyone. He rubbed the back of my neck, and then I launched off his shoulder and back into Sky. When I looked down, I saw him standing there looking up at me, smiling, for he was beginning to know how to read my thoughts.

8

Destiny & the Journey into Change

It was a full moon, and the cove was lit up like the Milky Way, colour and vibration everywhere. You could barely swim in Ocean, walk over Earth, or climb a tree without bumping into a representative of nature.

From a bird's eye view, it looked like a wonderland. Just off the Ocean, larger than anything around it, was Baobab, rooted deep into Earth. Surrounding it were oaks, sequoias, dragon trees, palms, willows, and the list went on. They were all rooted into Earth, that African earth, solid with a layer of softness over it. Scattered around the trees were flowers of every sort: roses, sunflowers, daisies, tulips, and so many more of every colour and shape. Then there were the animals, housed in, on, and under every tree. There were bees and dragonflies weaving in and out of the flowers. Ocean had settled itself into a bay, interrupted with a scattering of protruding rocks. Across Ocean and reclined against the rocks were pods, groups, and even solitary representatives of the marine world. Some lay on their backs, others moved up and under the surface like a sewing needle making their way across a material landscape. Every colour and shape you could ever imagine was represented and existed in perfect harmony.

We had begun to arrive earlier and earlier to listen to the story of our soulmates. Stories of torture, destruction of habitats, shootings, and cages, so many cages. Once in a while, there were stories of love, of how a human had saved them, freed them from nets left in the Ocean, traps on land, bought them back to life and then released them. Of how there were humans that walked beside them day and night in the African bush to save them from poachers. These selfless humans had dedicated their whole lives to us because they understood that their survival lay in us, not the other way around.

It was shameful in a way because they were protecting us from their own species. We would have had no need for them if they had learnt to live with us, to accept death, and to not constantly seek to prolong life to the point of even freezing themselves and regenerating their organs such that their population continued to grow to numbers that would soon be unsustainable. Why could they just not understand that death was life, not permanent but a transformation from one energetic life to another?

As I landed in the sanctum of the cove, I listened to a conversation in progress about destiny. A bee had been buzzing around a group of humans, who were explaining their present predicament and claiming that there was nothing they could do but surrender to their actions that were being guided by their destiny.

Before joining the conversation that was taking place by telepathy, I took a moment to take on the luminous glow of everything around me that was created by the light of Sun that had begun its slow disappearance as Earth rose. He used broad strokes to paint Sky with pinks mixed in with orange and a deep blue. It seemed all of us below it had taken on its hue.

"Eagle!" squawked Hawk, and I was shaken out of my transfixion of all that surrounded me. "Explain destiny to these bees would you? They have been buzzing around me with a question that I don't know how to answer."

"May I?" asked Orangutan, who was swinging from limb to limb greeting all the new arrivals as well as those that had been coming for months now.

"Why not?" I answered. I knew that Orangutan was a Yogi under all that hair. A slow-moving hush descended over the cove as all ears and senses turned to Orangutan.

"Hold on, wait for me, I want to know the answer as well." Out of what seemed like nowhere, Corey appeared. We had begun to feel so safe in this magical place that none of us had tuned into the approaching human energy. Most probably because it sat in peace and did not send out threatening or fearful signals anymore.

We all turned our heads in surprise as Moon rotated and Ocean swelled.

"Why hello, Corey." We greeted him in unison, and each of us saluted him in our own ways. He, in turn, placed the palms of his hands together and bowed back to us.

"You have become as smooth and slippery as a snake," said Snake, as his tongue whipped in and out. He made his way slowly up Corey's leg to wrap himself around his neck, hugging him all the way up. "See, humans keep mistaking my hugs for death squeezes," he sighed as he settled onto Corey.

Corey just stood there frozen. His mind was unable to comprehend that there was a snake wrapped around him.

"Corey, take a slow inhale starting from the expansion of the belly and then a long exhale. Close your eyes, drop out of your mind, and just feel Snake. Feel his warmth, his love, and, most of all, his humour. Keep breathing. Keep the exhale long, relaxing the belly in and up at the end of it. As you do this, remember that the diaphragm will squeeze the vagus nerve that runs through it and release acetylcholine that will kindly ask the heart to slow down its beat."

We all watched in silence as we began to feel the human's heartbeat slow down. By lowering and lifting the diaphragm, he gently moved his body out of fear and into awareness. In the place of fear, what we felt rise in him was joy as he surrendered to the energy Snake was passing onto him.

He opened his eyes just as his face broke open into a humungous smile, and he turned to look at Snake.

"Thank you."

Snake squeezed a little and then slowly made his way back to the Earth. Corey made his way to the edge of the Ocean, where I was perched on a hippo. There was no longer a need for words between us. Without a word, he conveyed his love to me and to all that had gathered and then sat down on Earth between a flamingo and an armadillo.

"Destiny," began Orangutan, "is another word humans use without fully understanding what it means. It is a word you throw around to excuse and escape responsibility for your actions, behaviours, and predicaments. Sadly, it is too often used to justify evil and meanness.

So, before we begin with the guidelines that are the foundation stones of Yoga, let me create some clarity in the amusement park that is your mind.

Now Corey, you may think it was a coincidence that we met, but there is no such thing as chance. Every single effect has a cause that is governed by the laws of the Universe, of which we all are a product. Therefore, our meeting was not by chance, but a direct result of a cause or a series of causes that can go as far back as our past lives. Everything that is happening now between us has a relationship to that which came before it and actions we took that delineated our journeys.

As you stand in your present moment and observe your life, know it has been defined by you and not by some force beyond you. You, yes you, have written the software that guides your life through the mental and physical habits you have created, through the neurological pathways you ride every day, through your repetitive thoughts, and through everything you give permission to enter your mind through your ten senses.

Basically, your destiny is influenced by everything you put in your mind, everything already sitting in your mind, and all the *karmas* and *samskaras* from former incarnations grooved into your consciousness. All these bear a tremendous influence on your actions, behaviours, thoughts, and words, and together they make up the software known as your mind.

This software determines the path your life follows. Every action you took at some point in the past is influencing your present life, and every action, thought, and behaviour you take in this moment will have an effect at some point in your future. And this will be your destiny, defined and created by you.

Now, fear not, because through the practise of Yoga you will learn that you are able to influence your destiny. This is accomplished by achieving mastery over your *koshas*, your body, your mind, your breath, and your life's energies. The last one is what leads to the absolute control over your destiny. With the others, you exert some control, however, your *koshas* still subconsciously guide you just like the software on your phone that is constantly running and doing what they have been programmed to do without you being aware of it.

Remember that your mind is vast, and there are hundreds and thousands of impressions that sit in it, all with the potential to influence your actions and hence your destiny.

Corey, all humans are vibrating energy, and that energy is full of information. The information that you vibrate inward and outward into the Universe will define the path you take not only in this incarnation but also in your future incarnations. And if you can control that energy, well, then you can completely control your destiny, including the form you take on in your next incarnation or no form at all.

By connecting to your Soul, your consciousness, to control or influence your destiny, you will also become aware of your life's purpose. Each one of us has a purpose, a part to play in the evolution of the planet or the collective consciousness.

Then there is the influence of all the other living beings on the planet whose actions in one way or another will impact you. We are all connected, so to change the destiny of the entire planet, it is not enough for just a handful of humans to clamber onto the path toward enlightenment. No, a vast majority of you must exit the merry-go-round that you ride every day and begin the climb up the mountain of knowledge toward your true self. And that my friend is the story of Destiny."

As Orangutan finished her grand speech, I looked around me to an orchestra of silent pondering. I was sure at some point a fuse was going to be blown in a cell somewhere. No one had really imagined just how complex the human form really was.

"And now, FINALLY, we shall begin to explain the eight limbs of Yoga, the toolbox that will get you to destination self, from which it's a hop, skip, and jump into the collective consciousness." I flew around happy as an Eagle could be to finally start laying down tangibles.

"Eagle, come on, let me start this story, pleeeeessse," squawked Hawk, flying around like a B52 bomber jet plane, except she killed no one but her food.

"Yes. Yes. Go ahead."

"Well, Corey," smiled Hawk with her whole body. "Scoot over a little and let me perch beside you. Ahh yes, much better; I love the smell of humans when they don't mask it with perfumes and soaps. Don't humans know that if you feed and hydrate your body well and look after it, your natural smell is delectable?"

Corey laughed at this, especially as it emerged from the most powerful hawk he had ever laid eyes on.

"Let us begin shall we? The first limb of Yoga is the ethical guidelines by which we live our lives known as *yamas* and *niyamas*. There are ten, which, if you think about it, is very interesting. Let me just remind you that Yoga proceeded all religions, and we shall leave it at that.

These guidelines are the foundation stones on which the yogic discipline builds the journey into the self. Therefore, anything not built upon this foundation is susceptible to collapse at any time. These ethical guidelines seek to clean and calm the mind, to cleanse the *chitta* and flatten the oceanic mind such that the *vittris*, the wave upon wave of impressions and thoughts, are not constantly rising to the surface. Once calmed and cleansed, the observer of all, the true self, can see its reflection in the purity of the mind.

Yamas are also known as abstinence or restraints and are five in number. They are *ahimsa*, nonviolence, *asteya*, non-stealing, *satya*, truthfulness, *brahmacharya*, moderation, and *aparigraha*, non-greediness. These are seen as great vows for all humans at all times and in all circumstances if that human seeks a life of freedom from all suffering.

Niyamas are five observances: *saucha*, purity, *santosa*, contentment, *tapas*, acceptance of pain but not causing it, *svadhyaya*, self and spiritual study, and *ishvara*, surrender to the Universe and selfless service to all living beings.

Now, before we go into slightly more detail about each, it is important for you to understand this: You can reach spiritual heights without embracing any of these guidelines, but there is a wee problem with this. Through the practice of *asanas*, *pranayama*, and meditation, you will move and shift *prana*. At some point, you will tap into what is known as the *kundalini shakti*, the divine energy that lays coiled at the base of your spine. When awakened, everything that is held in your mind, your tendencies, habits, samskaras, impressions, and thoughts, will awaken with it and be amplified. Therefore, if your mind is not purified and filled with tendencies toward anger, negativity, hate, sex, and greed, then this is what will be magnified in your mind. And well, I don´t think I have to tell you how destructive this will be not only to others, but also to yourself karmically.

Equally important for you to understand is that every time you engage in these ethical guidelines, you are planting seeds of love, kindness, compassion, acceptance, and truth in your mind. By repeating these guidelines in all your actions and words, you are then watering them until they grow into a beautiful mind. Every time you choose not to engage in a *yama* or *niyama* and instead choose to plant seeds of anger and other negativities in you, you nurture an unhealthy polluted mind. And might I remind you, Human, that your reality is based on your perception, which is influenced by your mind. Therefore, an impure mind filled with anger, lies, and negativity will create such a reality in your world as well as deep pain in your body because, as you will remember, everything gets stored in your cells.

I shall explain the first one to you today: nonviolence. This is kind of funny if you think about it because humans tend to only know violence. You rise to anger, you have violent, hurtful thoughts about others all the time, you watch it, you listen to it, and you eat violently as well. In fact, I believe that nearly every human has engaged in some form of violence or is exposed to it nearly every day, and you are not even aware of it. Violence, especially verbal violence often in the form of anger, has been normalized in your lives, in the shows you watch, in the music you listen to, on social media, and in movies, where anger with others and yourself is written into every script.

It does not matter the medium from which you absorb violence; the seed does not know whence it was planted. Your hippocampus, the hard drive in your brain, downloads every single thing you have exposed your senses to during the day, while your amygdala saves all your experiences from the day and the emotions you have attached to them. These then become the guidelines with which you interact with yourself and with others. When an event happens and you are too tired or stressed to think clearly and then respond, you will react. Your mind will scan through your hard drive and emotional centre for a reaction. It does not differentiate between fact, fiction, and fantasy. Therefore, if you have filled your data bank with violence, then you will react with aggression or violence because that is what sits in you.

Human, today be aware of everything you put in your mind. Of the music you listen to, the TV you watch, the people with whom you interact, the words you use, etc. How many contain some form of violence?

Then, of course, there is the violence toward one's own body in the junk food you eat. Although advertised as pleasure, there is only pleasure on its way down and then future pain from there on. And the worse form of physical violence to yourself, what other humans and media teach you, is that when stressed, you go to a bar, get high, drink booze, and have meaningless unconnected sex with people you barely know.

At some point, all those forms of violence become the influencers of your behaviours because they fill the storehouse of impressions planted in your mind. Most humans are not even aware of the violence they engage in every day. Did you know, Human, that every time you hit someone or say something violent to someone, you are hurting yourself? Literally. You are teaching yourself violence and moving your body into a state of stress. As you do this, the memory of violence gets stored in your body, albeit in your back, your hips, your ankles, or your wrists, and then creates pain. But more importantly, you are choosing a reality and life filled with violence because what you project out into the world is what your reality will look like, and what you project out will reflect what you put in.

Therefore, to be nonviolent means to consciously engage in non-violence and compassion on every level. When you feel anger, go for a swim or a walk and allow it to move out of you in a healthy way. See a spike in the road? Move it, so someone else does not get hurt. Be aware of the words that come out of your mouth. Choose forgiveness and kindness as responses to negativity and watch how magic starts to take place in your life. Every action has an effect that reflects the action.

But, do you know where humans are the most violent these days?"

Hawk paused here and stared deeply into Corey's eyes. "Well, do you?"

"In video games?" Corey mumbled, feeling like prey.

"Huh? That is not the answer I was seeking, but a good one because some of your video games are more violent than some wars that have been fought. I don't get how governments put so many restrictions and rules on humans, yet you are allowed to play violent games that teach violence to the player. And then they 'ooohh' and 'aaaahh' and wonder why there is so much violence in the world. But I got lost there. The answer is in your thoughts. I have seen a human meet someone, greet them, and be polite, and then turn around to say things in their heads like, 'I wish that person would drop dead,' or 'I hate that person.' Or you engage in violent thoughts about yourself with such statements as: I am such a loser; I am so stupid; I am not worthy of that person. When you understand that violence includes thoughts, nonviolence just gets a whole lot more challenging, does it not?"

"You got that Hawk," laughed Baobab. "It is at this stage that Yoga begins to weed out those who really seek change from those who want to play the video game of Yoga, wear the badge of Yoga, but not really practise Yoga."

"Now Corey," Hawk continued, "to end today's story of violence, let me squawk that when we speak of non-violence, it is not a negative thing but rather that in acting non-violently you are positively expressing the Universe that exists within you and which pervades in all living beings as love, peace, and calmness. The more you engage in nonviolence, the more you will become aware that the source of most violence in humans is fear and insecurity, both of which are fed to you from nearly every medium of media in today's world.

You know, Human, most of us in nature only sting, prick, or bite your species when you engage in violence with us or to survive whereas humans rarely use violence to ensure literal survival.

To begin the journey of non-violence, understand that it begins with the self-study of your mind and what violence sits in there. Here are some questions with which you can begin:

Are your thoughts and actions harmful toward others or yourself in any way? For example, do you put yourself down, say you are unworthy, or call yourself negative, violent words?

Are you careless or uncaring in the way you handle things or move through your life?

Are your dietary choices harmful to yourself and to other species?

Are your communication patterns non-violent? Do you seek to dominate the conversation? Do you listen fully to the other or do you get annoyed easily if someone does not agree with you?

Are you sarcastic?

Is your humour at the expense of other people?

How do you express yourself emotionally? Do you express yourself through anger, annoyance, or impatience? Do you consider the feelings of the recipient to your emotions?

As a beginner to this practise, you will fail monumentally sometimes, and that is okay. As you can see, these vows are huge. They are not as simple as not hitting a dog on the head or scratching letters into a tree's trunk, so set the bar low to start and create consequences for yourself every time you fail to engage in nonviolence."

Just then the air around us cracked open, and an enormous trumpeting sound reached into all our hearts and squeezed us so hard that our breathing became collectively erratic. I flew into the air and watched a herd of elephants come down to Ocean´s edge and crumble to the ground.

"What is it?" I whispered to the enormous African elephant.

It took him several minutes to lift his head. Tears streamed down his face. "They killed the females in our herd today and left the babies abandoned. They shot them, then tore their tusks out. They do not understand that to kill us for our tusks is like us killing humans for teeth just as killing rhinos for their horns is akin to killing humans for their toenails. And then they tell the human kingdom it has miracle properties.

They shot them in front of our young, who were left abandoned and traumatised. They took elephant lives to place our tusks on what? Mantle pieces, around necks, and wrists. Why? Why do we mean so little to you?"

He turned to ask Corey, whose tears mirrored Elephant's.

"Do you not feel pain when someone is violent toward you or does something that leads to the loss of your loved ones? Of course, you are so caught up in your mind and all the drama that constantly plays out in it that you cannot feel our pain. If you could, you would be crippled at the loss we feel. It is so large and envelops our entire soul such that our body weeps and with it the entire Earth. Our children are left feeling abandoned. They cannot understand where their mother has gone. It is no different from how your children feel when confronted with the loss of a parent."

He was not wrong. All of us, including the human, had felt the shift in Earth. It felt as if it would collapse at any moment, opening large black holes with no bottom and pulling everything in sight into the depths of its despair.

I landed slowly beside Elephant and placed my head against his. "I am so sorry, my brother. I know your pain; we have all felt it. If there is anything any of us can do, we are here for you."

Elephant raised his head and gently wrapped his truck around my feathered body. "Thank you. I feel no anger just deep sadness, and beside that sorrow sits forgiveness in my heart. It is only through the forgiveness of their ignorance that our healing will begin. I also understand from the conversations we have been having that the human will feel our suffering one day if they do not move toward love. I only hope it comes before they kill us and themselves off this planet."

I looked at Corey and silently motioned to him that it was time to leave. Although he was loved deeply by all of us, Lion and now Elephant were reminding us of the violence humans constantly engaged in with us. Even though he was different, he was still a symbol of that species. In this moment, we needed to heal collectively without him in our presence.

Before he left, Corey turned to the elephants and placed his hand on his heart. He sat down facing them and began to take long inhales and exhales. As we looked into his heart, we saw that he had begun the giving and taking meditation. He was imagining all the elephants' pain as millions of black dots slowly invading their bodies. With each inhale, he began to move the suffering up through their bodies and out of them, guiding the black dots toward him. He then took their enormous cloud of pain and inhaled it into himself and toward his heart. As it touched his heart, he turned the blackness into light, and then, in the next exhales, he sent that light filled with love back into the hearts of the elephants.

It transcended anything we had witnessed in a human. As we watched in wonderment, we could see a glow begin to radiate outward from the core of the elephants. Corey had begun the healing that we would finish.

When he opened his eyes, we knew that he was carrying the elephants' desolation with him as he began to walk away. I would not walk him today. We wanted him to carry our pain, to feel it, to know it. For only in truly knowing and experiencing our pain would he begin the path of transforming it into a pure love for us.

Once he was gone, we all sat and began an AUM meditation. In unison, each AUM filled with love moved our bodies. Even in our differences, we moved in synchronicity. AUM, AUM, AUM, AUM..............

9

Yamas & the Leopard

I arrived at the cove to find an audience captivated by a Black Rhino, who reminded us of an age when dinosaurs ruled our planet. She stood, a storyteller, sharing our history with humans. Their history books so rarely included any of us. But our goal here was not to change their history, but to add our perspective to it.

"My mother was named Baixinha by your species. She was an East African Black Rhino, one of 500 left in the world at her time of maturity. She was one of the unlucky ones, born in a zoo far from her home and all the space and distance we were meant to travel.

At some point, the story goes, she was taken to Brazil and from there to a celebrity ranch in South Africa. You know, Corey, she spent her entire life with your species. She was patted and fawned over, and then, after an entire life lived alone without a companion, a family, or familiar surroundings, her owners decided to can hunt her. The same thing that happened to Lions' family."

An audible collective gasp rippled across nature. All around the cove, mouths hung open, eyes rolled upward, and postures slumped over. Even Corey lay his head in his hands.

Rhino paused to take in the reaction to her story and allowed her listeners to process the fate of many of Africa's magnificent animals.

"As word spread across the hunting world, a Norwegian hunter stepped forth and offered 60,000 euros to murder Baixinha. An aware human and well-known South Africa movie star, however, saw all that was wrong with the hunt, stood up and saved her.

She took Baixinha, and with compassion and kindness, she found her a home on a reserve. There, she was loved and given the freedom she had never known but always yearned for. But alas, it was too late. Months later, she died. The stress and loneliness that humans had subjected her to had slowly worn her down."

As Rhino finished her story, what followed were moments of introspection. We all, including Corey, pondered on how we had gone from wandering the planet to so many of us caged and enslaved.

I quietly flew over to Giraffe and perched upon her head. It felt good to share our stories with a human as in those stories we were beginning to be seen and felt. It was the power of story to connect on a level where true change was possible.

"Welcome, nature. Rhino, thank you for sharing your story with us today and providing a different perspective to the Human of the impact of their actions on us such that they may understand that every time they cage one of us, they are, in fact, caging themselves into a world of violence."

We all bowed to Rhino to acknowledge her pain and tell her that we saw her. It is a beautiful thing to be seen. Then gently with awareness, we all shifted our energy to a place of gratitude and understanding that each of our energies has an impact on the collective.

I waited for the silence to move into *sattva*, and then I began:

"Take a moment to close your eyes. Be aware of all the sounds and energies that surround you. Know that you are not meant to be anywhere else but where you are at this very moment, so be here. Be present. Remember there is only this breath, this moment, which is life, so be in it, feel it, and embrace it. Now, gently rest your eyes on your heart and visualise a change that you desire. Imagine that it has come to fruition and sit in all the high frequency emotions, such as joy, laughter, bliss, happiness, that you will feel from it becoming your reality. Begin to pave new neural pathways from your heart to your brain. Teach your brain that this change has already occurred, thereby creating new habits, of high frequency emotions for you to ride in your body and brain.

Now, gently open your eyes and reconnect with your breath to move into the present. Before we enter the world of *yamas,* let me give you some human science. Corey, the heart is home to over 40,000 neurons and nearly 2 billion muscle cells. With these neurons, the heart speaks to everyone, including the brain. The flow between the two is predominantly between the heart and brain, not the brain and the heart.

When all your energy channels in and around your heart are unblocked, these 40,000 plus neurons fire in synchronicity and coherence. When this occurs, the energy that your heart gives off can literally be felt up to 10 metres away. Its electromagnetic field when tested with an electrocardiogram, measured 60 times greater in amplitude than your brain, even though the brain has nearly 10 billion neurons. The power of the heart to create change is greatly underestimated in your world. Now let us continue handing out your yoga tool box."

"Ahem," announced Leopard. "Let me get this one, Eagle. You know my mind is as pure as the river that runs through the mountains, except when I am chasing another species for sustenance."

I smiled at Leopard. Although he looked all violent, he was humble on the inside, and he was right about his mind.

"Sure, go ahead. Give my squawk box a break."

And so, he began:

"Human, the second *yama* is not lying. You would be amazed at how much humans lie. From the time you are born, you learn to lie from your parents, from TV, from friends. You are told lying is okay to protect the feelings of others and that lying is fine in some circumstances but not others. But this is not true. I believe there is only one acceptable lie and that is to save the life of another, literally. Any other kind of lie is just another layer that prevents you from reaching the ultimate truth.

When you lie, you cease to trust because you see your lies in others. When you lie, your body sits in the stress of holding onto that lie. There is also that common trap that all humans fall into when they find that lying about something brings about, for example, a financial gain and conclude that it is the lie that bought it about when really it was the effect of a cause that occurred long before the lie. If it were the lie, then every time you lied, you would have a financial gain. But humans don't see that part. The gain instead reinforces the behaviour of lying.

The lie that I find most amusing in humans is the giving of misinformation. When you don't know the answer to something, you lie and make up the information rather than admit that you don't know the answer. Do you have any idea how much harm you cause by doing this? Imagine someone who was bitten by a snake and in trying to fight off death follows the instructions given to him by someone who made it up rather than saying they did not know the formula. This seed of lying is so detrimental and the source of so much suffering and pain to yourself and others.

Seek to be courageous, to speak your truth, and to stop lying. Not all at once, of course, because you will fail monumentally at this. Maybe start by cutting down the number of lies you tell in day. Or maybe just start with being aware of how many lies you tell in a day.

'Honey, did you apply for a job today?' 'I did.'

That's a lie.

'Son, did you clean your closet?' 'I sure did.'

That's a lie.

'Babe, does this dress look good on me?'

Well, I think you are getting the gist here.

Here is a tip, Human. If you can't tell the truth, say nothing at all or tell the other you prefer not to say anything at all. You may be surprised how much time you spend in silence. Truth is wonderful. When you engage in it, it gives rise to trust and honesty in your interactions with other humans. Vast amounts of energy is freed up in you, and your truth gives rise to truth in others.

Lastly, the largest source of lies in today's human world is the gossip and frivolous conversation that holds no basis in truth that so strongly influences how you see the world. This laziness to not gain full knowledge ensures that most humans live a life based on half-truths and illusions and is also called ignorance. That is what gossip does: it breeds ignorance and suffering. Did you get all that Corey?"

Corey nodded his head as his mind began to move back through his day to identify how often he might have lied to others.

"Human, don´t worry about that now. There is no point in ever looking back unless it is to learn a lesson. You can start to observe your relationship with lies starting from this moment."

As Sun began to disappear, we stopped for a moment to watch Sky transform from light into a shining calmness. We observed how the colours reflected the change of frequency in the air. We witnessed and felt an orchestra being played out in colours and emotions as Sun played its last act before its show was over for the day.

"Goodbye, my friends. See you on the flip side," Sun saluted us. We saluted Sun back. Of course, we took it for granted that Sun would return the next day, but really who knew if it would?

"Now Human, the third restraint is not to steal. It is not as simple as it sounds because it does not merely refer to the theft of material, tangible things. Humans steal all the time, and you don't even realise it. You steal others' joy when someone gives you good news or retells a positive experience and you respond by giving them a similar story about yourself. You steal each other's time when you do not show or show up late. You steal other people's ideas, and, worst of all, you steal other humans' energy by dumping your baggage on them continually. Then there is all the stealing that goes on in your thoughts and in your mind, the always wanting that which belongs to another: 'I wish that girl would leave him and come to me;' 'I wish I could have her car;' and so on.

To not steal also means to find ways to give to others. It is in the act of giving that you are then privy to an abundance of receiving because the less you steal and the more you give, the more you will get back. It is that simple, really. Here is a game for you and your team to play this week when you get back to your world:

Give yourself 100 euro. Start to observe your daily actions. Every time you steal someone's time, energy, joy, positivity, love, or goods (and yes, that includes things in a hotel), deduct 5 euros from the 100. Every time you do something good for someone without the intention of getting back, i.e., just giving for giving, give yourself 5 euros. At the end of the day, see if you are in debt or credit. It may just surprise you just how much thievery you engage in without even knowing it."

Moon interjected, "Leopard, I think that is enough gardening for tonight. I have it on good authority that Corey is going to have to get back to his human world; a War is looming on the horizon. Wars are birthed through misunderstanding between humans, fueled by humans living in their desires and their reactive systems, and made of nothing more than pride, ego, and greed, all rising from that organ the mind." Moon's radiance dimmed a little, and we could feel the darkness that never seemed to fully leave the human world.

"Yes, Moon, I agree," moaned Earth, the element among us most affected by the actions of the human. "Humans do not understand that there is enough in this world for everyone to meet their basic needs, which is all one really needs. I mean, look at us, that's all we do: meet our basic needs and the rest is pure bliss. Well, unless a human is trying to kill us, capture us, or reduce our land to the size of a pool table.

Something's gotta give soon. This repetitive karmic cycle of war with just different players and locations not only kills humans, but also kills all of us. We are always the forgotten victims of war."

Corey looked across Earth. "I am exhausted by it and so much so that sometimes I can´t see the light until I get here and see all of you. You are the light at the end of a dark tunnel, all of you that exist around me and within me. I know light will come, but I also know that our species will have to hit the bottom of darkness to find the awareness to move into light."

"You are moving closer to it." I looked at the human.

"Come, let me walk you back. It will all be okay. This too, like everything else, will pass. The question is: what will it pass into? You know, Corey, you can change laws, alter institutions, win wars, and still nothing will change. Because changing those things doesn't change humans, whereas changing humans changes everything.

Because, let's be honest, humans abolished slavery, ruled against hate crimes, passed laws against trafficking women and kids, and, well, you know the list; you are a law man. But has any of that stopped? No, I thought not. Why? Well, because a human is still a human, and the mind is still the controller. To change that karmic cycle, humanity itself will have to change. And that, my friend, is where, if you just got it right, media and social media could be used to move all of you to the rinse, squeeze, and clean cycle."

Corey looked over at me, resting on his shoulder, as we walked out of the cove. "You know, Eagle, I have started to remove the boxes and labels others have put me in for so long, and you are right. It is so liberating."

"Isn't it just? I am glad that I don't fully know all the definitions humans have created for African Fish Eagle because I am not sure I could meet all those expectations. And what if I no longer wanted to be a Fish Eagle but behave like a flamingo instead? What would your lot say to me? That I could not because I am an eagle and therefore must remain one, behave like one, and never being granted the space to grow and move out of my box. I wonder, how do humans categorise a peahen who was born under the warmth of a duck and then raised by ducks? Is she a peahen or a duck? And does it really matter? And why should it matter, so you know how to behave toward it? And should you not behave equally with love and kindness to all beings, no matter their form?"

"Hahahaha, you have more whys than anyone I know."

"I do, and why not? It is the basis of self analysis. Now enough school for today. We have reached that point where we must physically separate."

I paused for a moment. I wanted to tell him how much I loved him and how beautiful he was to me, but I was not sure if it would be too much for him or if he would be able to receive it without creating a fear in him of losing it or being worthy of it. It did not matter how much I loved him. If he did not love himself and know he was worthy, he would not receive my love in the purity in which it was given. But to withhold it was to do insult to pure love.

"I love you, Corey." I spoke as softly as if I were handing him precious crystals.

He stopped abruptly and looked at me perched on a rock in front of him. I could see him blush and his mind racing. As expected, he was receiving it with all the filters of his mind rather than from his soul. I could hear the questions, the doubts, and the fears beginning to rise from the sinkhole of his subconscious to sabotage him.

"Corey, stop. Look at me. Close your eyes and focus on your breath. Let go of your mind."

I placed my wing on his broad soft chest. "Feel my love from here. Just feel. Just let go and accept it."

We stood there for minutes. On each exhale, I took light and love from me and passed it into him. As he softened under my touch, I sensed a crack in the walls and barriers he had built up to block out love. He placed his hand over my wing and, in that moment, we became one.

He slowly opened his eyes, and the blueness of his irises sparkled. I knew that, for a moment, he had understood what pure love felt like. I lifted my wings and flew off without a word. Last time we had left him with sorrow, and today I wanted to leave him with love.

10

The Enormous Restraints

I once flew across a place where they were hacking down trees as if they had no life in them. It seemed to be a common thread in humans. If something did not speak and could not articulate itself, it was soulless.

"I don't get it?" spoke Willow to nature's manifestations. "Humans are constantly campaigning other humans to not eat animals, to save the fish, but I rarely hear them say things like, 'don't buy wooden furniture,' or 'cut back on wooden doors and tables.' Where do they think all that wood comes from? I'll tell you from where: from my body and my arms. And once I am gone, I am gone. There are no prosthetics for me."

Willow chuckled at the idea of a prosthetic limb on this trunk.

"I hear you, Willow," came the deep voice of Dragon Tree. "It's like they know we are important, but they don't. A little like smoking: they know it can kill you and that it is bad for you, and yet they still do it."

"Hahahaha, you speak truths," affirmed Oak. "There is a reason that in the yogic discipline we are called the tree of life. Without us, there would be no life. For one, we absorb all the carbon dioxide humans keep ejecting into the air like a giant disco smoke machine. And then we give them back oxygen. We keep the planet cool. We help create clouds to protect the atmosphere. We remove pollutants from the soil and air. Our roots prevent soil erosion and floods, and we look dapper in all our various forms. I mean, I could go on and on about all that we do, but I know we must continue this story of Yoga because otherwise there is little hope left for us and, by extension, the human."

"It is true," uttered Baobab. "The human must learn that we are a large part of the puzzle of which they are a piece. Each individual human cannot keep going on as if their individual actions are so tiny that it does not make a difference. And yet, the individual's action and thoughts impact the entire planet just as cutting one of us down impacts the overall balance of energy. Can you imagine if a tree walked up to a human and said, 'We see that you have nine kids? You don't mind if we take one and turn him into a limb rest for me? For surely that loss of one will not impact your family.'"

All the trees in the cove were tickled by this, and, for a moment, they all visualised a life where they did to humans what humans did to them. But of course it was brief because not one tree engaged in negative thoughts, violent actions, or low frequency energy.

"It is because nearly eight billion of you think like this that we are in this predicament. I am telling you, Corey, change on a global scale starts with you, the individual human. Stop looking to others to solve the problem of the planet's demise. Instead look within you because there is so much power in there. Just the simple act of not using wood, recycling, and abstaining from excess materialism and eating resonates positively out into the world."

Corey was nodding this way and that way such that I feared his head would fall off. I landed on his shoulder, and I was happy to see he was comfortable arriving on his own.

"Sorry I am late everybody. Some human was trying to shoot me with a rifle."

"What! Why?!" Corey and a hundred other beings blurted out in unison.

"Well, I would love to tell you, but he did not seem to want to converse about it. But thanks to Corey telling me to zigzag were I ever targeted, I survived a bullet in my bottom, or worse, in my heart. I am sure he wanted to mount me in his house; he did not look like he was starving.

Yoga, Where the Impossible Meets the Possible

Give me a minute, will you? I need to lay down, find my breath, and use it to let go of what just happened. Holding on to something that is of no use to me anymore will only hurt me."

With that I lay down on the ground, closed my eyes, and began to influence my breath to slow down my heart that was pounding in my head. With each breath, I let go of what had happened and slowly moved back into the present. As I lay there, I began to smile. I could hear Leopard asking Corey about the zigzag thing.

"It is not as easy to target a gun as you may think. If it were, everybody would be a sniper," Corey sermonized. We were now in his expertise. "There are so many factors that go into shooting a target: your stance, your aim, your eyesight, your balance, and so forth. So, if you are ever being shot at, which based on what I am hearing at these meetings is fairly probable, run from side-to-side as fast as you can."

"Whaaaaaaaaat?" purred Leopard. "Why did humans not send out this memo at the beginning of time?" Leopard paced back and forth shaking his head until he came to a standstill in front of the human.

"Now Corey, let me give you some advice. If ever there is an animal chasing you, no matter which way you run, the chances of us catching you are pretty good." At this, he rolled on to his back, flipped all four legs into the air, and started laughing uncontrollably. And of course it was so contagious that all of us, including Corey, joined him.

"Thanks, Leopard." I lifted myself off the ground. "That is exactly what I needed to bring my energy back to its calm *sattvic* state and my mind back into the present."

Namaste, Moon, Earth, Ocean, trees, animals, plants, rocks, all of you really." I bowed to all those around me.

"Namaste," they all bowed back.

The Enormous Restraints

"Tonight under Moon, we shall finish the *yamas*. Please settle down onto your sitting bones or the part of your body developed to rest and turn your awareness and attention to this moment." I watched the Human lay down on his back and place his head on the belly of Orangutan. A connection had grown between them.

"The fourth form of restraint is abstinence, which does not mean a cease and desist order from all sex. It means to have restraint in your actions and to allow your sexual instincts to follow your mind and not the other way around. Thus, as your mind becomes more and more pure, your desire for sex will, in its own time, lessen. Because, let's face it, Human, if we asked you to give up sex all in one go, we would just be asking you to fail.

What is also meant by this vow is not to commit adultery because this is, by far, one of the most harmful things you can do to someone. That pain has far-reaching repercussions not only on the participants, but also on families, friends, and kids. Adultery also deeply affects those who commit that act by planting negative seeds in them. They find that for the rest of their life they continue to experience unhealthy relationships and that the search for a suitable companion remains elusive.

In ancient texts, sex was condoned between two consenting adults who had reached an age of responsibility so long as they had no commitments to someone else. In the yogic discipline, there is an explanation as to why humans are so deeply attracted to sex beyond procreation. In the human body, the main energy channel, called *sushumna*, runs from the base of your spine to the crown of your head. When energy flows freely through this channel, it allows for strong, elevated emotions to flow through it and can eventually take you to a state of bliss, enlightenment, nirvana, etc.

From the time you are in the womb, however, that middle channel begins to be choked from the side channels. These side channels begin behind your nostrils and run down the left and right side of your body to intersect the main channel in three main places: at the top of your spine, the mid-spine, and the lower spine (which is where humans often experience back and neck pain). These are known as *ida* and *pingala*. Not surprisingly, the human spine, nervous system, skeleton, etc., develops around and mirrors these energy channels known as *nadis*, of which there are over 72,000 in your body. In science, you would probably call them arteries, veins, capillaries, bronchioles, nerves, lymph canals, etc. It is intriguing how human anatomy reflects the movement of energy throughout the body. Even though *nadis* have no physical manifestation, there is an order to how they move through the body.

Your thoughts fly through these side channels, as well as your thoughts about your thoughts. They represent the duality that came out of creation of the feminine and the masculine. The left channel, *ida*, is the feminine, and is located where most of the nerves and pressure points for your parasympathetic system reside, the source of your energy expansion, the Yin in you. The right side, *pingala*, represents the masculine sympathetic side, grounded in the sun, and the system in which your unique creativity rises.

But I digress. When your side channels are flowing with positivity, kindness, giving, compassion, etc., your middle channel cracks open and you experience something akin to bliss. Humans can also feel this at the end of a good Yoga practise because the poses and breath work seek to open the choke points and let energy flow through the main channel.

You know that overwhelming feeling of love that sometimes accosts you, where you just want to explode? You know, like how you feel every time you are around me?" I exclaimed, teasing the Human.

"You feel as though you are floating and something in you has been opened, untethered, and released. That is what happens when the middle channels experience openness at the level of

The Enormous Restraints

the heart. In fact, when humans die, your side channels dissolve and the middle channel completely opens. This is why so many humans see angels, spirits, and light when they are dying.

There is another point, however, when for a moment, the spirit's breath flies up the middle channel and you experience extreme elation: when you orgasm. Yup, orgasm. And when you experience that fleeting feeling of ecstasy akin to enlightenment, you want more of that feeling. But like an orgasm, the feeling is temporary and does not create a lasting transformation in you. Yet humans chase it time and time again through sex, though never being completely satisfied because, like all emotions attached to desires, they are fleeting.

When you follow the yogic path, however, eventually you reach a point when that feeling of bliss and elation sits within you all the time once the desire for that fleeting orgasm wanes and you are unburdened from STDs, heart break, rejection, or the dumping of large amounts of energy.

The latter burden is one of the strongest reasons that yogis abstain from sex: to conserve energy that is used instead to fuel introspection and a state of internal joy. When sex is aggressive, fast, and unconnected, you lose energy with every orgasm as well as with all the negativity that accompanies such sex. That energy could be used to fuel your internal growth. Among yogis, it has been told that seminal fluid is a source of life that if stored properly and not ejected out into the world can bring forth vast amounts of energy. The same is for women who retain their orgasms. This conserved energy transforms into a subtle energy called *ojas*, which is often manifested as a magnetism or aura that flows off the individual.

Brahmacharya is all about not letting your senses and, hence, urges rule your behaviour because anything that causes turbulence in your mind gives rise to low vibrational emotions that drain you. Remember the game of 100 euros. If every time you had unconnected, meaningless sex just to orgasm, you had to give away 50 euros, would you be so quick to jump into sex?"

I took a moment to spread my wings and gave the orchestra of nature their moment to do so as well. For us, sex was not an issue at all. We used it to procreate and to ensure the survival of our diminishing species. But for humans, this *yama* was bigger than the tallest mountain and just as hard to climb to the top because it was deeply connected to their self-worth and their attachment to desires.

"Now the fifth, and last form of self-control in Yoga is to overcome possessiveness and attachment to things, your body, people, knowledge, money, events, and certain acts by not believing that happiness is to be gained by the accumulation of all the above.

For when you bind your emotional state to your attachments, you descend into a state of one of two minds. Remember the colouring of likes and dislikes? In the first mind, you find yourselves unhappy when you see someone else gaining something nice as if there were something so bad about someone else having a moment of joy because you think happiness should only be yours. As a result, you allow your mind to shift into envy and jealousy. Some of you even take it a step further by then stealing that other person's joy with gossip, theft of their idea, etc.

Walking beside this state of mind is the flip side, where you feel joy when another fails, tumbles into misery, and falls almost as if you are immune to catastrophe and it could never happen to you. What is wrong with you humans?! Really take a moment and observe yourself: How much of your day do you spend being unhappy at others' happiness and happy at their unhappiness because they either possess what you do not or have lost what only you should possess? Simply translated, this vow asks you to live without attachment to anything.

The Enormous Restraints

Because attachment, to your mind, your thoughts, your body, objects, people, places, is the root to all suffering. When you lose that to which you are attached, you suffer. Nonattachment, however, does not mean 'not caring.' Enjoy an experience. In fact, experience all the magnificence nature has to offer. Just don't attach your emotions and identity to it.

So, Human, please spend as much time as you want with us. We are always here to offer you love, but do not attach to us. We are not yours to own or to possess. Attaching to anything, including us, would be like a river attaching to a rock or a bank of earth. Imagine that."

I flew into the air and hovered. "There you have it: A place to start your journey and the foundation upon which we will now build. When next you join us, we will pursue the observances, and then off we shall meander onto the other limbs of Yoga.

I feel as if you all need a little rejuvenating, so to finish today's moonlit class, I kindly ask that those of you who can come into a headstand, a shoulder stand, or dive straight down into Ocean."

It was a circus worth watching as all sorts of appendages shot up into the air. In doing so, they gave energy to their immune systems, rejuvenated their legs, and lengthened their spines to give space for the nerves that shoot out of each vertebra. Each inversion aided their balance and gave rise to feelings of joy.

For some minutes, you heard nothing but breath and felt joy dance around the cove. The luminous human stood out among all of nature's beings for he was magnificent in his form.

"Now, slowly make your way out of the pose and into child's pose, allowing the blood to return to its regular sites. Stay here for a moment, expanding the back on the inhale and relaxing the chest on the exhale as if you were a bull frog." In one inversion pose, we had moved from the *rajasic* movement state to the *sattvic* calm state. Inversions are very powerful at creating that transition.

"Now, slowly raise your chest and uncurl your back vertebrae by vertebrae until your spine is elongated. Keep your eyes closed and connect with your breath to ground you back into the present. Place the palms of your hands together and thumb on your heart as we finish our journey today with our AUM. We begin our inhale now."

And just like that we merged again as it was meant to be: as one.

11

Butterfly Observes the Human

We had decided to meet during the day and on the designated human day of rest. It is so funny that humans chose a day to rest when really every day should be a balance between the active sympathetic nervous system and the calming parasympathetic system. They see sleep as rest, but sleep is very different from rest. In sleep, your body is still moving and your mind still working. They know that all energy seeks balance, and yet they keep forgetting that they are energy.

The human body is capable of carrying a human through every turmoil that ever accosts it. But only if it is kept in balance. If its ph-level, temperature, hormonal levels, etc. are maintained within a narrow bandwidth.

I had asked Butterfly to accompany Corey into the magical cove and answer any questions he had, so he could hear the same truths from more than one mouth. Sometimes I was not sure if he believed what came out of my beak. What we were explaining here seems farfetched to many humans. Which is why we were asking the Human not to take our word for it but to engage in Yoga and see for himself. It is not the Yoga that is challenging but finding the courage to change. It is so much easier to live in the addiction of suffering than to take responsibility for and a hold of one's own life and move out of victimhood.

Few people understand that trauma and bad experiences are not something that happened to you. It is how you process those events and then hold on to it. Holding on to the fear and shame of the events and then binding them to your sense of self.

So often when a human moves into a low frequency state, they apologise, claiming they do not know whence that eruption arrived. A human will often defend the act with the statement that it was not them. But it was all them. Every aspect of their behaviour is part of the mind, which is part of them. In denying the negative thoughts and actions that rise from themselves, they deny themselves change because change can only arrive when they are ready to accept and honestly see all that fills their mind by observing and accepting all their behaviours. It is only then that true healing and change are possible.

As I dove into the cove, there was chatter and laughter everywhere. A wonderful exchange of stories and energies was happening, aiding an understanding of the self through the understanding of others. Ocean spoke with Whale, Sun with the birds, Earth with the mammals, the flowers with the bees, and, well, there were more conversations than I could take note of. Amid it all sat Corey, just listening and observing himself. It was extraordinary to watch how he had moved from looking outside of himself for answers to observing himself and his interactions and into a place of self-awareness as he interacted with the world.

Through the sharing of stories, each of us was beginning to not only understand our fellow beings, but also ourselves as we were reflected in everything birthed by the Universe.

I landed gently on Corey's shoulder so as not to startle him, and he turned to me with the smile that melted me every single time.

"Hello, handsome Corey."

"Hello, beautiful Eagle. You look majestic today, as always. I hope that there is much more to this story. I am not ready to let go of all of you yet."

I rested my wing on his head and moved my beak closer to his ear. "There is some, but it too shall end at some point. Everything changes and transforms, and nothing is permanent but universal consciousness. But fear not, when this ends, it will transform into something that will reflect where all of us have moved forward in ourselves. For remember that our reality reflects us, so what all this transforms into will be reflections of us."

Corey pondered on this for a while and then smiled. He was beginning to understand that he had influence over his reality and it could become anything he wanted it to be.

"There you are, beginning to understand Yoga and its power."

"I am, thank you. To be honest, I am not sure I would have listened to this story from another human because, as you know, my trust in humans is very limited."

I fluttered all over and then whistled love out into the cove. In what seemed an instant, silence descended. Ahh, silence, my favorite song. I love silence. It comes with so much peace and clarity. I looked around, and everyone was sat in a yogic pose, their eyes shut as they began to move into the present moment. I could hear so many forms of *pranayama*, energy shifting breaths, being used to calm the heart and still the mind. When I began to speak, their full attention had arrived.

I waited for a few moments until I could feel everyone's energy, including the Human's, who now sat still on Earth with his back against Baobab's truck. And then I sent my thoughts into all of them: take a deep inhale, and, on the exhale, begin our three long AUMs. Each AUM was shifting our energy to connect to the energy of the cosmic Universe. Each AUM was reminding us that there was so much more beyond ourselves.

At the end, we sat in silence and in feeling.

"Hello, my beautiful friends. Thank you for being here. It is always a joy to enter a space where difference is revered and encouraged, where in all that difference, there is unity, respect, and, above all, love even though we all know that at some point in the future one of us may be eaten by the other for survival. Because it will be done literally for survival, we will not hold anger or animosity. Instead, we will understand that it is a part of the natural cycle of life and death."

I moved over to the elephants and perched on the back of the largest.

"Today, Human, my friend Butterfly, whose very being symbolises the transformation of life, will briefly explain *niyamas*. I say 'briefly' because each guideline is huge and time is not on our side. Our goal here is to give you the foundation of Yoga from which to launch you into change."

All of nature, of which Corey now saw himself a part, nodded and smiled.

Butterfly began to flutter around trying to find the right vantage point from which to project the large voice in the tiny form. In the end, she chose the top of Giraffe. I must say, those giraffes had been so gracious in lending their heads, always with love and never with resistance.

When Butterfly began, it was as if a bear emerged. Her voice was powerful and soft all at the same time. We all felt her voice move through us. It gently demanded our presence, which we did without question.

"Let me start today's lessons with a gentle reminder. Human, Yoga offers you the freedom to feel as free as we winged ones do and to remain calm amid chaos such that you can bestow calmness on others. In your serenity, others will be moved in the same direction. Have you not seen that when you smile at someone, it creates a smile in them? Joy, peace, and love are all contagious, and if you are going to die, why not die in laughter and joy? The practise of *yamas* and *niyamas* gift to you a life lived serenely.

The first *niyama*, gentle human, is *santosha*, the dedication to cleanliness mentally, physically, and emotionally. There are so many layers to this *niyama*. First is to have a clean home, office, Yoga room, and environment. Spaces that are not filled with clutter or draped in memories that keep pulling you into a past you tend to look at as an opium den of happy memories devoid of pain instead of serving its purpose: to teach you lessons. The more clutter you have around you, the more your attention keeps being pulled away from the present and from burning the unhealthy seeds that litter your mind.

Then there is also cleanliness of your body, the home of your soul. Feed it well, wash it, treat it with exercise, kindness, and sleep. Yes, sleep. Here comes that western science humans trust so much: Running like a river around your spine and brain is your cerebrospinal fluid or CSF. CSF not only drains out such toxins as dead white blood cells and other debris, but also acts as a bouncy castle that keeps the brain buoyant and protected from shock. During sleep, the brain shrinks and, through the process of osmosis, moves waste out of the CSF and into your lymphatic draining system. When you don't get enough sleep, there is a back up of waste that can lead to severe neurological diseases, like what would happen if you lived in a trash heap.

There has also been some talk in the medical field that lack of sleep and waste drainage are linked to the development of Alzheimer's. Sleep is also when all the information you have learnt during the day gets downloaded from your short-term memory drive into the hippocampus, your long-term memory drive, in your limbic system. So, the less sleep you get, the dumber you become. It is as simple as that. Lastly, when you don't get enough sleep, you move toward becoming a more reactive being by engaging in your emotional brain rather than with your calmer analytical frontal cortex, the *buddhi*. Thought takes energy, whereas emotion is the reactive tool of exhaustion.

One of the best ways to keep your mind clean is by not dumping layer upon layer of musical, TV, and Internet garbage into it, or worse still other people's negativity and fears. Be selective about what you put in your brain just as you are selective about your diet, clothes, hair, etc. It is a wonder anyone can find their soul these days with all the heaps of nonsense you keep injecting into your hippocampus and, by extension, your mind. More than any other interpretation of this *niyama*, the most important is to keep your thoughts clean and pure. Remember that thoughts travel and carry power, but they also exert influence over the body.

To purify the mind means to also release the baggage of victimhood and resentment that so many of humans insist on carrying everywhere. In cleansing the mind and the body, you lighten yourself. The lighter you become, the more fully you experience the magical mysteries of pure consciousness. Lastly, *saucha* is about being with each moment that arises as it is. Allowing it and yourself to be as is without wishing it would be anything other. Purity is about being pure in your relationship with yourself, people, work, the weather, and events as it is in the moment.

Corey, how often in your day do you just sit and put nothing in your brain and mind at all? How often do you give your mind a complete break? This is what you do when you come to your mat in Yoga, when you engage in conscious breath and meditate. The mat is where you allow yourselves to be observers of just how much nonsense is floating around in your mind and when you sit in purity with yourself unafraid of your thoughts and feelings, being completely open with yourself. Think: how often do you run away from yourself by always seeking some background noise of activity because you do not want to truly see yourself? There is so much liberation in beginning the journey of Yoga to purify all the toxins that sit in your mind and body.

The second observance is contentment through acceptance of all that is beyond your control. The first place you can start this is on your mat by accepting your pose instead of looking around the room and wanting it to look like the person's next to you.

Acceptance not only fuels contentment, but also creates space within you to change your own lives and for you to fill with thoughts of happiness, contentment, bliss, gratitude because you are spending less time focusing on the external and more and more on the internal. Seek to create contentment in your mind with thoughts of joy, courage, and healing. Contentment allows you to just be without seeking things external to you for happiness. Contentment allows you to not engage in likes or dislikes and to not force things. If something comes, let it come. If something wants to leave, let it go.

The third observance is self-discipline, or *tapas*, and doing something to the best of your ability. In Yoga, it is making a commitment to your practise even if it is 10 minutes a day. The basis of change, progress, and growth is mastering discipline and, at the same time, breaking habits. Discipline takes mental agility and effort, whereas habit is a laziness where you do the same thing repeatedly until it is something that your body does without the assistance of your mind. With Yoga, there is an enormous amount of discipline needed to meditate every day, to consciously observe yourself, to change your neurological highway, to teach yourself to be happy, to accept, to open, and to follow the *yamas* and *niyamas*.

In ancient scriptures, they see this observance as fueling the fire within you to know the self and to seek truth. In these scriptures, *tapas* is heat. It is to flame the fire within you to know yourself and to seek truth, so you may understand your purpose. One way in which this fire is fanned is by growing your ability to sit in discomfort and pain instead of burying or ignoring it in order to move through it with awareness and understand that you have to burn away the impurities in order to allow light to shine through and rejuvenate.

Corey, each of you are in the body you reside in, born into a certain circumstance, for a reason. Each of you has a purpose to move the evolution of this planet forward, and yet so few of you are connected to that purpose. We in the rest of nature live according to our purpose to maintain balance, but as you kill us that balance is being lost. In that void, there is human upon human all living a life completely disconnected from their true purpose.

Don´t you want to know why you are here?

The fourth observance is to study your self without judgement. It is the investigation into the unconscious patterns that govern your lives. We ask that you not only observe your thoughts, actions, and behaviours, but also your smell, your skin, tongue, and external self in order to be present in all your interactions. We ask that you not observe the other, but observe yourself as you move through your moments. In doing all this, you will be surprised at what you learn about yourself. You may not like what you see, but at least you will begin to see the layers and the boxes you have put yourself into that keep your true self from shining forth.

This *niyama* also asks that you study ancient texts and scriptures and find teachers to guide you and give you the tools to help navigate yourself and learn how to slowly erase all the layers that fog up your mind and drape your soul. This is not a journey that can be taken on your own. You need to have all the knowledge to know how to cleanse the mind, un-attach from the *koshas*, decolour your impressions, move *prana*, open your energy, and connect to your true self. For this you need teachers.

Deborah Adele in *The Yamas and Niyamas*, tells this story:

It seems the Universe had just created human beings. Realizing that he had made a terrible mistake. Universe called a council of the elders to help. When the elders gathered, Universe reported, 'I have just created humans, and now I don´t know what to do. They will always be talking to me and wanting things from me, and I won't ever get any rest.' In the story, the elders give all sorts of suggestions about where Universe can hide away from humans until one of them whispers in Universe's ear that she might hide herself in the human because they will never find her there. How true they were because humans always seek the answers everywhere but within themselves.

Now, Human, can I just flutter something here? How have you in the West allowed humans to take one Yoga course and then call themselves Yoga teachers? Are they not teachers of *asanas*, or maybe *pranayama*, and techniques of meditation? How many of those teachers truly know Yoga or live it? A Yoga teacher is a revered holder of great knowledge, one who never stops learning, who lives a yogic life, who teaches more than just *asanas* or breath. I sometimes fear that you have done to Yoga what you have done to love: trivialised it.

Now, the ultimate observance in Yoga, which you will no doubt understand, is surrendering to the Universe that pervades everything, including yourselves. You don't have to believe in an anthropomorphic representation of God to accept that there is a divine design, a benevolent essence in the Universe. There is no such thing as coincidence, chance, or miracles. You are connected with the infinite space the surrounds you. Therefore, if you can trust and surrender to it, it will surprise you time and time again. And get this: it is accessible to every single human without baptisms, rituals, or customs … All you have to do is start to climb the tree of Yoga limb by limb.

Let me end with this. Corey, life is filled with suffering for it is suffering that drives you to *tapas*, the search for your true self. Suffering fuels the flames of change and of desire for a life without suffering. The journey of Yoga is not to keep you in suffering but to teach you to live above it and to move through life with peace and calmness."

In ending, she bought her wings in and took a bow as nature erupted into joy. Corey, however, remained still. He had already begun to take a journey within to explore his connection to these observances. It was then that I noticed he had bought the bag filled with candles that I had requested.

"Butterfly," I began, my voice resonating as strongly as Butterfly's but at a different frequency. "Thank you for that master oration. So simple and yet not. Now loving beings, please bring you ears, eyes, nose, feel, and mouth back to me. I have a treat for you today, if someone can shake Corey out of himself."

Cheetah, who had arrived that day, gently stalked over and raised his front legs onto Corey's shoulders, so when Corey opened his eyes, his first thought was, 'I am going to be eaten here.' Some seed no doubt planted in him by some TV show.

"It's okay. Just breath," whispered Cheetah in his best, 'I am not going to shred you to pieces' voice. "I am not going to hurt you. I am merely hugging you, so I may have some of that human love you have been passing around and in return give you some of mine. This means I am not just hugging you to give you love. I seek to receive it as well, so could you kindly wrap your arms around me and hug me back?"

That schoolboy nervous smile we had all learnt to love was back, and Corey wrapped his arms around Cheetah. Each squeezed the other, and, in turn, each of us felt the love rise and embrace all of us, so much so that we all turned and hugged the being beside us. Ocean hugged walruses; animals hugged trees; bees hugged flowers. It was my ultimate dream come true.

Touch, especially hugs, is important on every level through every species. It connects us in a way nothing else does. It transfers love and energy in a medium that is not marred by the mind, fear, or filters. It was pure, and it was powerful.

I laughed as Elephant hugged me with his trunk and I hugged back with my wings. We did not speak. Instead, we were completely present in the hug as our energies were greeting each other and exchanging love. It was not a case of one receiving and the other giving. We both gave and received. It was how love in its pure energetic form is meant to look like in every relationship. A hug is a hug not a noncommittal pat on the back to aid the other with so much distance between the two huggers that another animal could fit between. No, a hug should establish a connection of love between two souls. A moment of silence, when each hears and feels the other and each takes on the others' pain, turns it into love, and returns it. It is by far my most favourite form of giving and taking.

And so, we all hugged in silence. It was incredible how much could be heard in silence. It is where the Universe existed, and in its vibration, shakti, creativity, and consciousness sprung forth. It is where existence came into being. Therefore, it is in silence that our consciousness, our soul can be heard.

We all gently let go, reluctantly. We watched as Corey lit all the candles that he had placed around the cove.

"Well, my friends, normally we would each have a candle, but that is impossible. We would need hundreds of candles, so we shall do my favourite thing. We shall share. Now, I know none of us need to teach our brain to focus on one thing, but I thought it would be nice for Corey to have some company in this meditative exercise.

This is how this works: Stare at one of the candles without blinking. When your eyes begin to water, which cleans them by the way, close your eyes and hold the image you see between your eyebrows for as long as you can. When the image disappears, open your eyes and begin to stare at the flame again. The image is often round, has colours, and possibly a dot in the middle. How long the image remains depends on how long you can focus.

No, Hawk, it is not a competition, and there is no winner. Now Moon, if you don't mind, can you turn your light down for a little while? This is best done in darkness."

"Ahh Eagle, I love your unending faith in my powers. How about I just hang behind a cloud for a bit?"

"Fabulous, you are a genius." I smiled up at Moon, the celestial splendor to which I was so deeply connected that when it was full, it pulled what we were all truly feeling to the surface for us to explore. If it could move oceans, rise tides, and lift waves to great heights, then surely it pulled all that lay within us. After all, we are mostly water.

"Okay, nature, yes, Human, you as well, shall we begin?"

And thus, a different silence from the one created in our hugs descended upon us. This one held calm, peace, and gently nudged us into ourselves as we began to shut out the external world and take a deep dive into ourselves.

12

Masculine & Feminine: Bigger Than a Penis or Vagina

I arrived after class had begun and was elated to see that the students had become the teachers. I landed softly on the top limb of Baobab, made my energy as quiet as possible, and listened to a starfish explaining the masculine and feminine to Corey. This was appropriate for Starfish had started its life's journey with male reproductive organs that were transformed into the female organ at maturity. Starfish embody what we all are: forms seeking to balance the masculine and feminine that exist within all of us.

"Now Corey," narrated Starfish from the rock on which it was perched. All its arms splayed in a perfect display of texture and colour.

"Let me first explain that the terms 'masculine' and 'feminine' are human labels defined mostly by one's genitalia when, in fact, they are forms of energy that have nothing to do with genitalia. But for teaching purposes, we will continue to use the masculine (Yang) and feminine (Yin), which exist in the gross level of everything.

Let us begin with the concepts of 'I,' the 'soul,' and 'me,' the mind or personality at the level of the cell. Now listen carefully. An atom is composed of electrons that revolve around each other vibrating at a high degree. The formation of an atom is from the clustering of negative (feminine) electrons around a positive (masculine) proton. The positive influences the negative to behave in a certain way to give rise to an atom. When we speak of masculine and feminine, we are not speaking of your sexual weapons but of vibrations. Note also that in this context there are none of the connotations humans normally attach to the terms 'negative' and 'positive.'

It is in the negative (or feminine) node, pole, etc., that new forms of energy and creativity are designed. A feminine electron or 'corpuscle' (which is a tiny particle) naturally leaves a masculine corpuscle and seeks union with another masculine corpuscle in the journey to create new forms of matter/energy. As the feminine vibrates rapidly under the influence of the masculine energy, it creates a new atom manifested in new ideas, creativity, and the expansion of energy. Although, the new atom holds the properties of its creator, the masculine centre, it also has its own individual properties.

Remember that if the Universe were Shakespeare and all of us his characters, then each of us would be a creation of Shakespeare. Each of us, however, would also have our own essence and character as well. Put another way, without Shakespeare there would be no characters, yet each character is not a direct mirror of Shakespeare but a distortion. In humans, the creation of new atoms at the cellular level mirrors this.

The feminine is the active creator, but only by working off the male energy. Therefore, what it creates is different from its creator but holds the same properties. Thus, everything in the organic world contains and manifests both genders. There is always masculine in the feminine and vice versa just like the concepts of Yin (feminine) and Yang (masculine).

In Yoga, when we speak of the 'I,' we refer to the soul that resides in all living beings. When we speak of the 'me,' we refer to the conditioned mind and, by extension, the conditioned personality. Each is influenced by the polarity and rhythm of emotions and the movement of *samskaras*, experiences, impressions, and thoughts. For some, the 'me' extends to the external physical self, which they then bind to their personality (i.e., their clothes, their looks); they cannot imagine a self that exists independent of the body. The self that is independent of everything is the 'I'.

The 'me' is where all your ideas, emotions, thoughts, and other mental states are housed and created, also known as the *chitta*. The 'me' (the feminine) needs energy from the masculine 'I,' the soul (remember the atom's creation), to generate new ideas and thoughts, either from the I, that resides in oneself, or someone else's I. Please take note that the 'I' (soul) may also recline back in awareness and objectively observe the creative process because although generated from it, it is independent of it.

The feminine 'me' always moves in the direction of receiving impressions, and the 'I' directs itself to giving. The 'I' gives rise to will, and the 'me' gives rise to creation and imagination. But if you are not connected with the 'I' in you, lazy really, then the 'me' will happily receive ideas and thoughts from external sources instead of producing original mental creations generated from the will and energy of one's own 'I.' This is why humans are so susceptible to the thoughts and ideas conveyed by clever marketing, charismatic people, TV and social media and why they so easily take on the ideas of others and make them their own. It is for this reason that we ask you humans to witness what is yours and what you have taken from others and convinced yourself is yours when you observe your mind.

The fire of *tapas* has yet to be flamed in many humans to connect to their own soul. Overwhelmed by life, constantly on the move, they have little time or inclination to do the work required to connect to their true self. Instead, most humans would rather take the words of others as truths than seek the truth within. In that context, are you a follower or a leader?

Will, when awakened in the soul, rides on the river of thoughts. Each gives birth to unique creativity that is positive and evolves all consciousness closer to light. When you live through pleasures and desires, however, will gets buried and submerged by the mind. Only by purifying the mind and un-attaching from one's desires does will flourish through the power of thought.

Human, there is nothing that is impossible in the world when pure thoughts are driven and transmuted by the will of the soul. For example, Corey, when you give up the habit of drinking Diet Coke, you do so by first controlling the sense of taste. By destroying a *vasana*, which is an impression that influences your behaviour, you are eliminating a craving by decolouring and burning a seed of like.

In that freedom you gain from breaking a negative habit, there is some peace to be gained. The energy that was once spent craving a particular soft drink is now converted into the power of will. With this newfound power, you will continue to overcome other cravings. In doing so, you will feed your internal willpower to lead from your true self and true **I,** not the egocentric I, thereby purifying your mind and connecting you to your true purpose, to give rise to the unique creativity that lays within you. Human, you will know when this will is blossoming within you for your eyes will sparkle, you will move with a magnanimous gait, fear will have fled, and a magnetic and dynamic personality will arise from within you.

Will is the soul. It is the infinite void of silence that pervades everything. As the feminine electrons vibrate around it, it gives rise to *shakti*, the vibrating aspect of consciousness. It is in this vibration that existence was given birth. This dynamic between silence that pervades all and the vibration that reverberates out of it to create is in every human. Therefore, what limits you is not your soul, that is limitless, but your senses that keep you bound to the external and the constant recycling of the same ideas.

Your attachment to the gross forms of masculine and feminine limit you as well. You don't see that these two polarities exist in unison in each human and are constantly seeking balance with the other. When you feel love, you do not say that you feel masculine love or feminine love; you just feel love. You are not male or female, not Indian or American. There is no us and them. You are just conscious energy interacting with matter (nature), seeking balance, creativity, and evolution.

You are powerful beings in your own right. You do not need someone else to empower you. Power that is given to you can also be taken from you, and that power thrives on the weakness of others. True, authentic power does not require the subjugation or weakness of anyone. To access this true power, the feminine vibrating, circulating energy in each of you, you must connect to the silent introspective conscious will that is your soul. Only then can you experience a power that does not constantly seek validation from all the resides externally to you.

I know, Corey, that you are wondering how one begins to access this power. Well, besides all the other tools we will begin to lay at your feet, you can meet your power by unblocking your *chakras*.

I will be brief here. This topic is as large as Yoga itself, but I shall crack open the door and add to the foundation of knowledge that we are building for all humans. Please know that this really is the tip of the iceberg; the topic of *chakras* is as enormous as those hippos lounging at the edge of Ocean.

The word 'chakra' literally means 'wheel' in Sanskrit and symbolises the flow of energy in your body. Although there are thousands of energy channels in your body, known as *nadis*, these seven main centres are where large numbers of *nadis* congregate.

Each *chakra* is like a world unto itself, with its own brain, functioning systems, endocrine glands, and influencers to the overall functioning of your body and mind. It is also the place where consciousness meets the body, in other words where mind meets matter. When balanced, consciousness may influence your emotions and physical lives in a positive way and lead you to feel connected to something greater than yourself. When blocked, consciousness is unable to flow uninterrupted, and you the human are left untethered like a pinball bouncing from one place to another.

I, personally, like to imagine *chakras* to be large concert venues. When opened, they are filled with vibrant, happy, dancing *nadis* celebrating life. When closed, a *chakra* resembles a graveyard.

All seven *chakras* are housed along the main energy channel, *sushumna*. Your lower *chakras* are deeply connected to *shakti*, the feminine creative force about which we have been speaking. The root *chakra*, *muladhara*, is located at the base of the spine with your gonads and where your fundamental identity lies, the ego self. It is the seat of fear, the place where you explore who you think you are. When this *chakra* flows uninhibited, you understand that you are not the content of your life but space, the silence in which the content exists. You are not the effect; you are the cause.

The second *chakra* is known as *svadhisthana*. The sacral or sexual *chakra* is located three inches below the navel. It embraces the ovaries, the digestive system, and the pancreatic glands. It is here that your childhood resides and issues that you have with yourself and all the things to which you have tied your sexuality.

As these two chakras come into balance, you find yourself feeling more complete, grounded, fluid and creative. The third *chakra*, *manipura*, is located behind the naval region below the rib cage and hugs the adrenal glands. It is associated with self-confidence, self-discipline, and wisdom. When balanced, you know who you are and can let go and live without resistance. You no longer engage in self sabotaging behaviour.

From here, you slowly move into the more introspective will *chakras*. The fourth *chakra* is *anahatha*, also known as the heart *chakra*. Located behind the breastbone, it is here that you connect to the cosmic consciousness from the dive board of love.

Next there is the throat *chakra*, *vishuddha*, home of your thyroid gland. It is from here that you express your truth in your thoughts, your words, and all the roles you play in your lives. As you travel further up, you arrive at *ajna*, the third eye *chakra*, which embraces the master pituitary gland. When in balance, you become a more resolved human who is self-sufficient and can connect to your inner source of happiness and bliss.

Masculine & Feminine

Lastly, there is the crown *chakra*, *sahasrara*. The seventh *chakra* is also known to be responsible for the direct connection between you and the Universe via the pineal gland, the antenna within your body.

So, you see, Corey, you are more than just your penis or your vagina. You are both male and female, the manifested forms of energy. To take the spiritual journey, to come into your own power, you must embrace and balance both masculine and feminine within yourself. You must also allow for the uninterrupted flow of energy throughout your human form.

You are living in a world right now that is very masculine heavy and creatively dull. Men are seeking to hold onto their masculinity, and women are embracing theirs. As a result, the feminine creative force is being subjugated, and the planet as a whole is imbalanced."

Upon finishing, Starfish inched its way into the water and disappeared.

"Well, that was a surprise," I chuckled, "but a much needed one. At some point, we were going to have to explain those concepts to you. I am happy Starfish decided to take on that task today and threw in the seven *chakras* as well."

Corey was still staring at the Ocean bewildered by Starfish's sudden disappearance. "Is it returning?" he asked me.

I shrugged because that was all I knew.

"Ahh, okay, well if Starfish comes back when I am gone, please thank that well balanced masculine and feminine being for today. I can't believe that all this is Yoga. All my life, I have overlooked Yoga. I thought it was something I should do if I wanted to tie my shoes without falling over as I got older. But this, the magnitude, the science, the knowledge is, well ... I can't find a word that accurately describes my total and utter awe at what you, the pure unsullied manifestations of the Universe, know."

"Why thank you, Corey, and I shall pass on your love to Starfish. Now, I would like to change direction just a little here and move into thoughts and emotions. It is too late to start the story of *asanas*, so, if you are okay, may we can talk about emotions?"

"Well, umm, yeah, I guess so. As you may well know, we men have recently been dumped into the garbage box of being emotionally unavailable. This makes me laugh every time I hear it because it is not that we are emotionally unavailable to others; we are unavailable to ourselves. All my life, I was told not to cry, to hold my emotions in, to control them. Even now, I am told by friends both anatomically male and female that when they cry they are told to stop. Don't even get me started on love. We men were taught that love is an act and not necessarily an emotion. Fix the car, buy a washing machine, build a swing, but do not actually express love. Our mantra is *be strong, courageous, and brave*. Everything else, bury and resist such that when we do engage in emotions, what follows their expression is the emotion of self-loathing for having them."

The empathy in the air was palpable because under that luminous exterior we had all witnessed the war of emotions that was continually being fought in Corey.

"Let me take this one," emerged the gentle voice of Baobab.

"Corey, let us move backward to move forward. Come sit here on my limb. There are several perspectives and layers to emotions, and each of them is connected.

First, according to the ancient Hermetica texts, a pendulum of emotions constantly swings back and forth in all humans, from happy to sad, fear to courage, calm to anxiety, etc. It mirrors and follows the movements in nature: the tides, the Moon, the Earth, and all the other planets. Its motion is like your breathing, autonomous and beyond your control but not beyond your influence.

Each set of emotions, although opposite in your experience of them, exists on the same plane. You can imagine it as a seesaw, with one emotion on one side and its opposite on the other. The only thing that separates the two is the rate of vibration. Both exist on the same piece of wood. When you are vibrating faster, at a higher level, and energy is flowing through you freely and openly, the seat carrying happiness will rise to the top and vice versa. But of course for this to happen, your organs and glands must be functioning properly, which is where Chinese medicine enters.

In Chinese medicine, at its simplest explanation, each emotion is attached to an organ that is also connected to one of the five elements that exist in all humans. What emotions rise in you depends on the health of an organ. The kidney is connected to the water element and fear. The liver is connected to the wood element and anger. The heart is connected to the fire element and joy. Now, please know that emotions do not arise merely because of the state of an organ. When there are extreme movements in an emotion, however, this is often associated with an imbalance in an element and thus an organ.

In today's sedentary lifestyle, the human body has become very misaligned. Because of this, the organs and glands are no longer sitting properly in the fascia and no longer function efficiently, giving rise to a chaotic cocktail of emotions. Which, as you now know, leads to humans attaching thoughts to those emotions, which then translate into unhealthy reactive behaviours. This is what we animals like to call the internal human domino.

However, the opposite is also true. The rise of emotions is strongly connected with your mind. Your thoughts have a direct influence on your glands that release such hormones and chemicals as serotonin, dopamine, and cortisol into your system. These give rise to emotions, which in turn affect the efficiency of all your organs and systems. If the emotions are negative and low in frequency, the workings of your organs and systems will slow down. In turn, that will encourage the low frequency emotions to stick around longer. It is a bit of a chicken and egg that one.

Do you know, Corey, that when you live in negativity and stress, you fuel negative emotions that then dump nearly 12,000 harmful chemicals, called peptides, into your body within a timeframe of 90 seconds to two minutes? These chemicals block your cells from absorbing nutrients. If this is a fleeting emotion, then the harm is negligible and the cells become unblocked. If you stay in this state and bury the emotions, however, then the damage is long-term. When your cells die in the state of stress, news ones are created in their place. Each new cell will arrive with receptor sites for chemicals related to negative emotions rather than for absorbing nutrients. This, of course, is a very simplified version of the whole process.

Then, of course, there is the energy of eight billion humans that resonates out into the world and affects every living being in its path. A world where the vast majority of humans are ejecting negative thoughts and words out is not a good thing for your species, which is then not a good thing for us. Add to this the traumatic energy rising in the world from the slaughtering of the rest of us in nature every single day, and you begin to understand the forces that keep you struggling. Well, unless you practise a discipline such as Yoga, which teaches you to live in a state of bliss and peace in the internal jungle of emotions.

Corey, I am going to say this again: humans have the power to change the world and yourselves just by changing your thoughts that influence everything from the cell upward in you and in every living being with which you share a planet as well. Ever notice how when someone negative walks into a class or a room, it affects all the people in that space? Your companion's negativity can create an unhealthy change in your own emotions and in your body because thoughts have power.

I know we have spewed out a lot here, so let me pull this all together for you. All organs and glands are connected to *chakras* and the movement of energy, so when energy is blocked by negative thoughts, misaligned bodies, poor breathing, etc., *chakras* cease to flow uninterrupted and all the organs and glands in their sphere malfunction. This gives rise to some low-frequency emotions, attached to by some negative thoughts, giving rise to unhealthy behaviours which in turn dims your life force to leave you feeling more like Darth Vader, dark and heavy, rather than Yoda, the enlightened one.

Therefore, Human, emotions are fabulous because when observed objectively they can tell you so much about yourself. They tell you where you are malfunctioning and where you are stuck. Let me make this easier for you. Let's say you are feeling insecure, and it is beginning to make you feel a little nuts.

First, sit in silence or go for a silent walk in nature and just listen. Don´t think or analyse anything. Just listen to your breath, to nature, and what rises from the silence. The source of that insecurity lies in you and most probably has a history. If you just listen, you will learn whence it comes. That is, if you are honest with yourself and don't play hide and seek. Often you don't want to hear the truth because in knowing the truth you will have to make a change that you fear or speak a truth the consequences of which you are unsure.

Also, be aware that if you are tired, not eating well, not drinking enough water, if there is a full moon, you are on your period, or there are large shifts happening on a planetary scale, these have an influence on your emotions. Take note if you are so exhausted that you are sitting in a reactive state rather than a responsive state because this will also influence your emotions. Remember, Human, others do not give you emotions. You give them to yourself.

With that in mind, observe the thoughts you have attached to the emotion. What is the source of those thoughts? When strong negative emotions rise in you also check what organ the emotion is attached to and see if you are treating that organ well. Make a note if you are practising yoga or any other discipline that opens and moves energy in you or if your body is all misaligned and blocked because this too affects your emotions.

Basically, take a journey of awareness into yourself because emotions are always telling you something about you. It is just a matter of whether you want to hear it or not.

Whatever the source of the emotion, it is of utmost importance that you hold space for them within you. So that they can move freely through you and out of you without resistance. You need only begin by accepting that you are not your emotions. That you are merely a conduit for their expression to teach you something, and then move through you.

Too often humans hang onto low-frequency emotions, attaching to them and not wanting to let go of them because you have identified yourself with them. They become a part of your identity as the person who is always sad, complaining, negative, happy, etc.

The more you attach to emotions, the more they become habits and addictions that are hard to break. For some of you, instead of trying to break the habit, you find comfort in it. You make excuses to stay in them because in them you don't have to do the work to change. Or even worse, you feel guilty about being happy or unworthy of happiness because you have convinced yourself with that powerful conditioned mind of yours that you deserve to be miserable.

That is why it is so important to let unhealthy emotions go once you have learnt the lesson they are teaching you. The longer you hold on to them, the tighter they will hold onto you.

Once you acknowledge that emotions are teachers, however, you understand there is nothing wrong with expressing emotions in a healthy way. When I say healthy, here are some examples of what I mean: Speak to a friend; go for a walk; take a swim or a run; write it down; sit in meditation and just listen; or put it in an audio and listen to it. Do not drink, smoke, shout, rise to anger, or any other act that is negative and detrimental to yourself or others.

What is unhealthy is burying them, resisting them, pretending you are okay when clearly you are not. When you do this, they will eventually manifest themselves as a disease, uncontrollable anger, self-harm, an addiction, or a number of other negative behaviours."

Corey stood up and started to pace, climbing over animals, avoiding swinging monkeys. "Excuse the interruption, but what you are saying is that I must learn to hold space for my emotions, to stay present in them without attaching to them because emotions too, as all things impermanent, shall pass. I must learn to live above the pendulum of my emotion, by sitting in the stillness that lies beneath it all. It is in this stillness, the silence between breaths, the quiet that pervades everything, that I can witness everything clearly, including the source, and accept everything as-is rather than to react to every emotion."

"Bravo! Bravo!" nature hooped and hollered, dancing the uncontrollable dance of life.

Baobab smiled, and we all smiled with her for Corey was finally understanding that Yoga was not something that you did but something that happens in you. It is a disappearing act into something beyond physical boundaries, impressions, emotions, and ideas and into the silence from which sound and existence were birthed. In Yoga, there are tools that labour to bring humans into alignment with the cosmic energy, and it is only when all is aligned within them that their total absorption into their soul is possible. How liberating it is for those humans who were truly able to see themselves from the platform of their consciousness.

"Corey, I believe that today you felt Yoga. Now, before we disperse, shall we salute the Moon with our moon salutation and offer up our intentions for this new moon cycle?"

Before any of us could answer, Baobab raised her limbs to Moon, paused, and sent out love to the space above. Then, on her exhale, she folded forward, dropping all her limbs' residents onto Earth and some into Ocean. It was raining nature as every tree in the cove instinctively followed suit.

As we landed, we got up, dusted ourselves off or swam to shore, in some cases aided by a dolphin. We then lined up behind the trees and moved with the trees and plants in their half-moon salutation. When we were done, we had successfully moved all the varying emotions out of us. We lifted our hearts to Moon and AUMed three times, each time holding the silence at the end to allow for our vibration to connect to everything around us.

When we were done, chatter erupted, and I flew to Corey.

"Are you ready?" I asked amid a rock show of joy and laughter.

"Not really, but I know I must return."

I whistled and silence dropped like thunder over us. I turned my head to Corey and nodded.

"Thank you again for explaining the masculine and the feminine in me today and providing me with knowledge about my *chakras* and the tools to start observing my emotions from a place of non-attachment. In every conversation, I am beginning to find joy and peace within me, and I have finally stopped searching for it outside of me."

With that, he bowed, and we all bowed back.

And just like that, the lightning of joy struck the cove, and they were all back into life.

"How have you been?" I asked Corey as we meandered back to duality, the world where everything was perceived as separate.

"I am feeling challenged. You have opened something in me, a deep desire to know my true self. You are right about the hard work. I thought my job was hard, but this path is bigger than any challenge I know. Meeting this one will make every other challenge a ride on a cloud."

I laughed with him, and then there was silence as we watched the other and listened to how that felt within us.

"You pass through my mind often. In the beginning, it was hard, and I suffered with the distance. But in time, it has become easier. I know I only need to sit in silence to hear you and feel your thoughts that are always filled with love. I am beginning to understand this thing called 'love' more clearly. We humans toss it around all the time as if we know what it is, but really most of us have no idea.

I was thinking the other day about how we are always asked to fight for the love of our country, to work hard for the love of our family, to toil and sweat to earn our happiness. In all of that, what gets sacrificed is love. We hardly spend time with our loved ones, until one day that love diminishes as we have invested in everything but actual love. That includes loving ourselves. We are never asked or told to take time to love ourselves. Love our job, our country, our religion, our cars, our lives, but never ourselves."

I landed on his shoulder and lay my head upon his. "You are becoming wise through awareness my friend. You are right. Humans claim to be the champions of love in all their acts, but when it comes down to loving yourselves and spending time with love with others, you fail monumentally. As for us, you are the twin to my soul and no matter where this journey may take us, you and I are connected for eternity.

And one more thing. Corey, choose happiness and peace in your thoughts, in your actions, and in your behaviour. Forgive yourself for whatever it is that is preventing you from being content with yourself. Learn the lesson that needed to be learnt, and then move forward. Imagine what a beautiful planet we would all live in if all the energy moving around was being propelled by high-frequency emotions."

Corey rubbed his hand over my head, pulled my head closer to his cheek, and then he turned and kissed me gently on the side of my beak. It was as if I had been struck by electricity. For a moment, he lingered there, and I allowed him and myself to stay there. Inside, my smile extended across my whole feathered body because I was witness to the impossible meeting the possible.

13

Yoga Asanas: Getting High Off Your Own Body

As its simplest explanation, the brain is the mechanism through which the mind operates. The mind is the mechanism through which consciousness expresses itself. Consciousness holds all the impressions and samskaras *from your present and past incarnations. Using the tools of the mind to clean and purify the conditioned consciousness (*chitta*) enables you to reach pure consciousness (*chit*). The body is the vehicle for all of it. Consciousness pervades the whole human form as energy not just the mind. The mind is just the washing machine for consciousness to purify and see itself. The body and breath are vehicles for consciousness/energy to move freely throughout the form, pervading every cell and system, so they may operate to the will of pure consciousness, known also as your soul. The will of pure consciousness seeks to create balance, peace, and joy, all the way down to the cellular level. Once attained, consciousness then uses the entire human form to experience life and express its will from a place of non-attachment.*

As I glided toward the cove, I was beginning to understand that there were so many problems in the world: slavery, poverty, mental illness, disease, suicide, violence, depression, hunting. I could probably spend an entire day reciting all the ills that plagued the world as it stood today, especially those facing children.

And yet, the root and solution to every problem begins and ends with the human. And not just any human, the grown human, who without breaking their karmic cycles, unbeknownst to themselves, then gives birth to another human onto whom they then pass all their luggage, thereby ensuring that the karmic cycle of their suffering continues in their children. Most humans are unaware that the foundation of the children they germinate into life is primarily influenced by their behaviours, thoughts, and actions. Ask any aware, enlightened human what they have uncovered as the source of their suffering, and the answer would most likely lie in their childhood. Therefore, where humans really need to start to create change is with children. If humans wanted to survive and not destroy the planet in the process, they would have to raise a generation of children who love themselves and engage *yamas* and *niyamas* from a young age.

I knew Yoga was enormous, but there is a place where every human can start the journey whether they be an adult or child. That place is the mat. The underrated mat would be the star of the story today. There would also be a surprise narrator, that many humans were very connected to, just not in the way we wanted them to be.

I dove into the cove with a full belly and used the air to carry me to that place of magic. I was excited to see that telepathy was still working its wonder. Every morning and every evening, I sat in silence and bought my wings together over my heart. I then began to visualise the Human and send him thoughts of love. It started out with the Human, but over time it had extended to all humanity. I understood the power of my thoughts and the energy that they carried to great distances, and I also knew most humans are weak and succumb easily to suggestions. Knowing all this, I used the power of thought to send love out daily, hoping to override all the nonsense they take for truth and all the negativity they keep feeding their minds.

As I arrived in the cove, there was a radiance that could not be touched but could be felt. We had become a meeting place where we all felt safe and where collectively our energy and our thoughts were creating shifts on the planet. Our individual power was collectively exploding into a light so powerful that it was touching all of nature across the planet.

I greeted Ocean and its residents first, then Earth, Sun, and finally all the other energetic beings. I scanned the landscape and found Corey swimming with a shark; a sight I knew I would see one day.

I turned to the whistle function in me and began to whistle a tune to allow for a gentle settling into silence. As Corey emerged from the water, I nearly choked on the air being ridden by my tune. We had become so used to seeing humans in clothes that their natural form was a bit of a happy shock for all of us. Once humans had openly shown their form and had sat comfortably in their bodies. Religion had covered it up and, in doing so, had sexualised it.

I wondered whether if the Universe had created each human to have multiple colours, as it had in the rest of nature, would the human world look a little different? Would it have been harder for humans to use their definitions of black and white, dark and light to segregate the human species?

As silence was uncovered beneath all the noise, just as our soul showed itself as the mind quietened, I watched Corey saunter over to the elephants and lay his back against them. He had put on clothes, much to all our disappointments, because he was uncomfortable in his own form. I was not sure if he was moving to a place of deep connection to us or if we were conditioning him to believe he was one of us.

As we settled in, Cow, Rooster, and Pig arrived. In a way, they were our ambassadors; they most often featured in the human world just not the way they would have liked. We all understood the eating of each other to survive, but the average human ate three meals a day and often in quantities that were above and beyond survival. When they did, they were unknowingly engaging in violence. They were killing.

"Welcome my fellow beings. As always, I am humbled by the trek you take every month to learn about the human. Today we welcome Cow, Rooster, and Pig as we begin the journey into asanas."

We watched as all three of them made their way to Corey and sat down beside him. They knew that every day he ate one of their species and not just to survive.

"But before we begin, Corey, there are some terms you should understand. The autonomous nervous system has two well known branches: the sympathetic and the parasympathetic nervous system. There is a third system, but that is for another day. A human's sympathetic nerves are at the core of your survival system, i.e., the fight or flight response. They spring from the middle of the spinal system at the first thoracic vertebra 1 to 12 to the lumber region, 1 to 3. The system evolved to protect humans from life and death situations, which no does not include deadlines at work, plumbing issues, relationship woes, and all those other events that humans falsely treat as life and death situations.

It was meant, for instance, for when one of us was chasing you. Now, when this happens, your analytical brain goes for a beer, your emotional brain goes nuts, and all your blood goes to your extremities. For example, your eyes dilate and reduce your peripheral vision, so you can focus on your attacker. You begin to crave sugar because your body wants that sugar for your muscles, thereby putting a halt to the absorption and processing of sugar by your cells. All the happy bees, as I imagine them, that work on your digestive, immune, and regulatory systems stop working, pick up spears, and head for your extremities to prepare for survival.

But worst of all, your body starts to dump cortisol from your adrenal gland, which in the long-term results in diabetes, digestive problems, memory loss, high blood pressure, weight gain, and a drop in your immune system among a host of other ailments and diseases. Human, when your body is under constant stress and it believes that it is at war or being chased by a shark, all the above takes place. When this happens, your vibration lowers as your cells, organs, etc. are not getting enough oxygen from your shallow and rapid breath. Your systems stop working efficiently as the bees go to battle, and you get stuck in low-frequency feelings of fear, anxiety, depression, anger, and irritability among a host of other emotions.

Please know that your sympathetic system is not all bad. There is a fabulous activation of this system when you take long or rapid inhales during moments of good stress that releases adrenaline and not cortisol. When this happens, what wells from the depths of you are unique creativity and positive energy.

Now, your parasympathetic system (PSNS) is your calm healing system and the state in which everything works as it should, without you having to go to an opium den to induce relaxation and calmness. In this system, your analytical brain, your *buddhi*, can operate from a place of awareness. This system slithers out from the medulla in your brain and the sacral region of your spinal cord. It is linked to your exhale, and when activated, it tells your body that there is no external threat and that all is safe and good. When this happens, all your organs, glands, and systems can work at 100% to heal, rejuvenate, and restore you. It is in this state that you can switch on or off your genes, specifically those linked to genetic diseases. When this system is activated, you are immersed in feelings of calmness, peace, kindness, and gratitude.

Now Corey, as we meander along this story, we will go deeper into these systems. I find it helps humans to know what is going on in their bodies when they practise the limbs of Yoga."

"Yaaa," erupted Hawk. "Very important stuff here. Few humans understand the body that carries their soul. It is amazing how you walk around all day not knowing your own machine and expecting someone else to fix it when it falters. One day, Corey, you must tell us why it is that so many humans just don't want to know themselves."

Before Corey could answer, Cow turned to him and asked in this softest moo, "Yes, Corey, hello, good evening. Maybe you could also tell me why humans enjoy eating me and my friends here just for pleasure. I have no doubt that if one of us ate you for pleasure, we would be shot."

"Weeell," stuttered Corey, "it's because you all taste so good."

There was a collective gasp in the cove. For a moment, we all stared at the human as if seeing him for the first time.

"I was joking. I am so sorry, but it is the truth. Humans eat you because you taste so darn good."

"Well, well," oinked Pig, who had been rolling on the ground scratching an itch. "You would not mind if I took a bite out of you then? I mean, I am full, and there is really no need to, but hey, I am willing to try you for pleasure."

Corey looked up at me to save him. I just shrugged. There are consequences for every word, thought, and action that rose from him and into the Universe.

"Ahh Pig, stop messing with the Human," cackled Rooster. "It's okay, Human, he ain't gonna eat you. You don't factor into our survival that way, but it would be nice if you understood that we have souls, feelings, and are living beings just like you just in a different form."

Corey bowed his head in surrender. Pig came over and kissed him while Cow licked his face and Rooster did a little cock-a-doodle-doo dance around him. Corey melted into laughter and knew that he would never again look at the meat on his plate the same way.

"Okay. Settle down you two. Get your face off the Human," doodled Rooster. "Eagle has asked me to begin the story of *asanas* today, even though there is no rooster pose. Not sure why that is; I am a fine specimen of strength and flexibility," he exclaimed as he did a little line dance on the earth to the amusement of all.

The cove settled down, Ocean calmed its surface, and Rooster expanded his chest and began:

"*Asanas*, when taught correctly, are a journey into Yoga. Each pose challenges you on every level to accept, surrender, and move energy and to slowly work your way through the poses that challenge you the most to observe all that rises to the surface in those poses.

Although *asana* practise is just a small part of Yoga, in today's world it has become important as the human body stagnates from sitting in a chair or a couch for large parts of the day. In

Yoga Asanas

the Yoga *sutras*, *asanas* only hold but a few pages. I believe this is because way back in the day humans were more active and healthier. Today, few humans sit in contemplation or meditate as their bodies do not allow it. They suffer from back and neck pain, inflammation of the joints, and a build up of toxins from lack of movement and poor diet. It is for this reason that we will spend a little more time on *asanas* than was originally set out in the Yoga *sutras*.

Asana literally means a seat, so a steady comfortable posture. *Asanas* prepare one´s body to sit in the stillness required for meditation. In conjunction with breath, focus, and the use of *bandas*, which are the locking of limbs to direct energy in a certain direction, the physical practise of Yoga aims not only to remove toxins, sluggishness, and laziness from the body, but also to energetically open the flow of all 72,000 *nadis* or energy channels by removing blockages and bringing your body's energy back into alignment with the cosmic energy. *Asanas* create the strength and flexibility to meditate without your body constantly pulling your attention and energy to it as it screams, 'get me out of this sitting position.' Each *asana* also massages the organs and glands in the body to keep them working efficiently.

The blockages I speak of in the body are the mounds of negativity that you humans ingest daily because you do not understand that thoughts and emotions block energy in the body and leave it feeling heavy.

The mat is also a place where a human can begin to remove the *kleshas*, the coloring of your impressions. In every pose, you should observe what rises to the top of your waking consciousness as you open your body and release all that is buried in every cell from your connective tissues to your muscles. Once observed, you should let go of it and return to your breath. Every time you choose not to give energy and attention to anything negative, you are starting to burn those seeds and moving them back to neutral.

At its basest level, *asana* practises start to bring your body back into alignment as if you were straightening out a rolled up, twisted hose to allow the energy to flow uninhibited through you. So many of your human bodies are twisted and out of alignment these days from sitting in front of computers, mobile screens, steering wheels, and TVs." Rooster demonstrated this by sticking his head between his legs. It inspired giggles across the cove.

"With the use of breath, you push energy through you in a calm rhythmic manner rather than sporadically or fanatically. With each full deep inhale, you stimulate your good, sympathetic, energetic, creative nervous systems, and with each complete exhale, you ignite the calming, healing, parasympathetic nervous system. This brings your nervous system into balance and prevents you from harming yourself.

You cannot and should not start an *asana* practise when you are angry and stressed because the harm to yourself will be grand. Low frequency emotions increase the tension in your muscles, which leads to chronic contractions and spasms. This occurs due to a lack of oxygen and blood supply to your muscles. When this happens, you begin to see an increase in lactic acid in the muscles and blood. This chemical then sprints to the brain to tell it you are stressed, which then increases the tension in your muscles even more, resulting in muscular pain, strains, etc. This is why in Yoga you should start any practise with breathing and awareness exercises to calm and quieten you before embarking on the physical journey of *asanas*. It is also why you are always asked to visualise sending all the oxygen you are inhaling to the area you are stretching or strengthening.

Asanas truly are a dance between your breath, your body, and your mind. You inhale to lift your self, giving your muscles and joints the oxygen to lift you, and exhale either when you move downward to relax your muscles into the stretch or when strengthening to remove all the carbon dioxide and stress from the muscle. This slowly allows all that is buried in your cells to be set free. To do this, you must be present and aware in every movement and pose. Only then will you gain the full benefits of a Yoga *asana* practise that is fundamentally different from just stretching.

Understand that muscular contractions, like how your shoulders are always trying to hug your ears or touch your chest, are massive energy suckers. They reduce blood flow, increase inflammation, and reduce the intake of nutrients by your muscles. It's why sitting hunched over for hours is so detrimental for your health. As your body contracts and your breath becomes erratic and shallow, the diaphragm has no space to lower and expand. Therefore, only the top part of your lungs has space to move, and this leads to a dramatic reduction in the flow of oxygen and blood to your entire body. This sends your mind into a tailspin and affects the release of such hormones and neurotransmitters in your body as serotonin, cortisol, endorphins, norepinephrine, and dopamine, all of which serve to increase your immune system, your emotional, mental, and physical health, and, most importantly, your sanity.

After calming the mind with the breath and bringing it in to the present, most *asana* practises begin with sun salutations. These are guided and coordinated movements with your breath. Each salutation moves your muscles and joints, increasing the flow of blood and oxygen through your body as well as feeding such parts of your body as your spinal discs and joints, where there is little to no direct blood flow such that only through movement and osmosis are they fed.

The body is the starting point for the meditative journey into yourself. Therefore, when you practise yoga *asanas,* here are some things to be aware of: Your body should feel firm but comfortable. There should be no tightness, tension, or discomfort; you should be able to comfortably stay in an *asana* for a length of time. There is a good chance if that is not happening, that your ego is performing the pose and that you are engaging in your mind and not your breath. When this happens, the entire benefit of the practise will be lost on you.

While in that slightly uncomfortable, comfortable pose, your mind should be focused on your breath. For example, by holding each pose for five breaths, counting up to four on the inhale ,and back to one on the exhale. Appreciate each pose as an opportunity to train your mind to focus on one thing. Lastly, the breath should be constant, the inhale matching the exhale as it flows smoothly throughout the body.

Yet there should also be a sense of freedom within a pose to move and adjust within the following boundaries: The skeleton, especially the spine, should be locked and aligned, and the joints locked into place. There should be no grinding or pain. You should avoid sitting directly on the earth because the earth is a conductor of energy, and unless all nine of our energy losing holes are closed and your *bandas* locked, the energy you are unlocking will seep out of you.

Those nine holes are your ears, nose, mouth, eyes, anus, and genitals. It is also important that *asanas* are practised in a clean space, devoid of any stimulus that may draw your senses and, hence your energy, outward. Cows, goats, beer, music, and swimming pools are no-nos. Such practises should be called something other than Yoga *asanas*. In addition to this, humans should practise in a place that is neither hot nor cold. The aim is to minimize sensations that draw your mind and, hence, your energy. Where your attention goes is where your energy flows.

The whole practise is about not only accepting the limitations of your body, not judging your body, being kind to your body, but also understanding that you are not your body. Surrender to a pose, especially one that challenges you, to know that all you can do is breathe through it, accept it, and know the limitations of the asana is beyond your control in that moment. What is in your control, however, is your breath and the knowledge that, in time, the poses that challenge you the most will be the ones you come to love because you will have taken a long and inspiring journey through them of learning unattachment, surrender, acceptance, and letting go."

"Rooster," I gently interrupted her flow. If it is okay with you, can we stop here today and Orangutan will pick up the story at the next full moon? It is getting late, and I thought we could end with an AUM meditation.

Rooster stopped prancing, and all three of them exclaimed "Yaaaaaaa" in unison. As really, compared to all of us, their suffering was enormous.

I knew Corey felt uncomfortable, and that was good. Discomfort, like emotions, is a flare sent out by the mind that something needs further investigation and change.

"Okay. Find your meditative positions. Make sure your spine is elongated, your jaw and face are relaxed, and your eyes are resting on your heart or third eye. We will do seven As resonating from the chest, seven Us vibrating through the throat and seven Ms emanating from the head, followed by seven complete AUMs. Please follow my pace and rhythm so that we are all in synch. By being present and aware, you may in this meditation begin to feel your form disappear into vibrating energy."

And so we began. Words could not describe the sound and the feeling of connectivity to everything. The bliss and energy that arose out of us collectively was magnificent. There were no words, and therefore I used none.

14

Asanas Practised by Orangutan

We had all decided to arrive at the start of the new moon. I had gotten word that today hundreds and thousands of fireflies, also known as lightning bugs, would light up the cove for us. Now come on, really, the Universe is genius. You only had to look at all of us in the cove and our internal mechanisms to witness the Universe's creativity. The human body is a work of art. Its mechanisms and systems are more advanced than a space shuttle. Everything that a human needs to heal, to live a healthy beautiful creative life in perfect harmony with its environment, exists within them.

And yet they just keep building concrete structures that have no life and are devoid of any integration into the rest of nature. Sure, some few had built eco-structures that were not intrusive on us, but for the most part so many of us had died and then been replaced with non-energetic concrete, air conditioning, and processed air. Each city is bringing the planet further into imbalance as its energy source disappears. Humans are literally choking the planet, and its slow death is being manifested in fires, hurricanes, earthquakes, and other acts that try to bring the planet back into balance and to bring back its breath. It is so desperately trying to heal itself, and humans do not see that.

We all knew that there are many among them who want to live in balance with the rest of nature. Society, however, has made it such that only the well-off can afford to be environmentally conscious in their decisions. The average human in today's world cannot afford the cost of living above plastic and in eco-friendly homes. Why is healthy food and healthy living so unaffordable? Why is junk food, booze, cigarettes, plastic, disposables etc., so affordable? Why do they not heavily tax the latter to subsidize the former?

But it was, what it was. All we could do is change the present to influence the future. And what a present it was! The cove was lit up by thousands of twinkling lightning bugs. Had I not known where I was, I would have believed that I had arrived in outer space with its trillions of dancing and singing stars as I arrived at the end of the journey. Hypnotized by the splendour, I thought the end of every journey should look like this. And maybe it did, and we just cannot remember it.

I found Corey by the water's edge cooling his feet in Ocean as the heat and the humidity rose all around us. He was deep in conversation with a loggerhead turtle. I smiled. I knew Turtle's story would amaze him, and yet he would probably miss the point that all that wonder existed in him as well. He just had to connect with it.

The loggerhead turtle weighed between 180 and 300 pounds, some weigh up to a ton. They begin their journey by emerging from the sand with hundreds of other babies that slowly make their way back to Ocean. Only one in a thousand survive that exodus.

Destined to never know their parents, they begin their journey across Ocean with only the love and knowledge of the Universe to guide them. Seventeen years later, with no GPS system or Google Maps, they are guided by Moon to find their way back to the place of their birth and to give birth to a new generation. With all the knowledge that lives within them, they know how to dig a hole with flippers the size of a human leg that does not collapse and houses up to a hundred eggs. They know exactly how to cover the hole without killing the eggs and to show no trace on the surface that they had ever been there. They know all of this, and yet no one sits down and teaches them it nor do they attend turtle school.

Loggerhead turtles are content in their solitude, only mixing with males to gather as much sperm as they can to fertilize hundreds of eggs over a period of three months. To all of us, they are remnants of an age of dinosaurs. They are magnificent, and they too are in danger of disappearing, like the dinosaur, as the humans hunt them for pleasure eating. We excuse the very poor ones who do so to survive, but not those who eat them for pleasure or to sell them without understanding that they are eating part of their own consciousness. They are eating themselves out of a planet, out of life. But it is not just the feeding of humans that is killing them, so too do the nets in Ocean and all the artificial lights on the land of their birth. These white lights leave them so confused that they often got lost and die, unable to find their way back to the Ocean.

I landed beside Corey and greeted both of them.

Corey turned toward me with a sparkle in his eyes. I could see the child in him emerging as if he were truly seeing the world around him for the first time. How important it is for adults not to lose that child in them.

"Hello, Eagle. Did you know … Of course you know. The story of Loggerhead here is mind blowing. How they know where and when to come back, guided by Moon, the stars, and themselves. And they are so warm, loving, and peaceful."

"I did know all that, and did you also know that the moon calendar is etched on their shells? In some native Indian cultures, it is believed that the turtle is the holder of all knowledge. They are also one of the longest living species in the world. Some can live up to 150 years."

Loggerhead moved a little closer, allowing Corey to touch her face. As he did, he leaned in and gently kissed Loggerhead on the cheek. "Thank you for sharing and for allowing me to see the soul in you and the power of the Universe. I am so sorry for what my species are doing to you."

Loggerhead bowed her head. "A time will come when it will be too late to see us and to see that we too carry joy, give birth to life, sustain the planet, and have a soul. Too late to see that we

Asanas Practised by Orangutan

love and suffer just like you. In our case, the human is often the source of our suffering, whereas in humans, you are the cause of your own suffering.

It was a pleasure to feel you, Human, to know the kindness and compassion in you, and to connect to the soul that you are still seeking within. I have seen what you cannot: your purpose. It is my deepest hope that one day, through Yoga, you will connect to your true self. Only then, will you really know and see us."

With that Loggerhead turned and gently slipped into Ocean, a place they had all once felt safe, but no longer. In fact, there was not a place on this planet that was safe for us. Not the earth, nor the skies, nor the waters. Even in places where there are no humans, humans impact our lives because everything is connected.

I left Corey deep in thought and flew up to the top of the Baobab. I was humming softly as I did. I wanted to give everyone time to settle down and ponder on their own brilliance.

"Hello beings and lightning bugs. Today we sit in gratitude for the luminous light you provide us in a world with much darkness. Orangutan, dance your way over to the Human and bring him to Baobab as we continue to teach him the benefits and necessity of *asanas*."

Orangutan swung her way over to Corey. We all watched in amusement as she danced and shimmied over to Corey, took his hand, and led him back. We saw the joy move back into him as Orangutan swirled around him. She was also humming a tune of happiness.

She settled him onto an arm of the tree and began as the rest of us lay down or reclined into ourselves and listened under a blanket of stars up in the sky and their reflection in the fireflies that hovered around all of us.

"Human, let's talk a little more about the human spine. It is one of the most important structures within you. It lays over the main energy channel, *sushumna*, and houses two nerves from every vertebra, which is the switchboard of the human body. Although there is blood supply to the spine and vertebral column, there is no direct supply to the discs. This is similar to the joints and ligaments that only through movement and compression get fed. No movement and no compression mean that you are basically starving the connective tissues responsible for holding your human forms together.

Therefore, when practising asanas, the spine should always be straight -- even when you are bending from the waist (unless you are intentionally seeking to work the back muscles). When the spine is straight and elongated, the central and peripheral nervous system, which sprouts from it, are neutral. This means they are not being squeezed or stimulated to send a message to a body part that then draws your attention away from your breath. A straight spine instead allows for the smooth flow of energy, known as *prana*, through them. If the body is twisted in a way it should not be, then the flow of energy is disrupted.

Yoga *asanas* are so not an exercise because you should find a stillness in them that is swayed gently by your *sattvic* calming breath that frees you from the polarity of opposites that enslave humans: hot-cold, hunger-thirst, joy-grief, etc.

When you achieve harmony in a pose between your body, breath, and mind, your metabolic process slows down and is calmed. This, in turn, lessens feelings of hunger, thirst, and other desires, all of which act as agitators to your energy. At a cellular level, your cells begin to dance because there are no threats to which it must attend. Instead, they have time to construct, heal, and reproduce. Rather than depleting your energy, they create energy. At the same time, through rhythmic inhalation and exhalation, your emotions are calmed, and blockages to energy are broken down. This is why you feel so darn good after a Yoga *asana* practise. It is also why you begin to feel subtle shifts within you as your energy begins to vibrate and resonate at a higher frequency.

Now Human, there are so many variations of *asana* practises that it is hard to know what they all mean. Many of you, without proper knowledge, attach yourself to one type of practise and stay there. In that sense, *asana* practises reflect how humans live and limit your lives. You get addicted to one type of practise. You work on only one part of the body, mostly muscle, and ignore all the other parts of the whole: your joints, fascia, bones, mind, organs, and breath.

So today, Human," swung Orangutan off the tree into a somersault and onto the ground, "I am going to explain the different masks of *asanas,* so you may practise with knowledge not ignorance."

She began to move around and every so often came into a warrior pose, as she began to narrate:

"The different practises you so often hear about are mostly a way of sequencing poses. In Yoga, there are historically a set of poses that open, stretch, and strengthen your entire body. As Yoga has moved to the West, the *asana* practises have become more flamboyant with the introduction of an array of new poses, each aimed at keeping the student engaged. Yet, the point of yoga is not to mentally stimulate you but to disengage you from your mind by repeating the same traditional asanas such that you can move deeper into them and gain all the benefits from each.

Yang Yoga practises focus on muscle and stimulate your circulatory and lymphatic systems. The latter is an important network that flows from all your tissues and organs to your lymph nodes. There, it picks up white infection immune cells and filters out such foreign material as bacteria and cancer cells, which like all good visitors should eventually leave. It collects excess fluid from tissues and cells and returns it to the blood stream that was too full to accommodate it, and it absorbs fat from the digestive tract. As you can see, the lymphatic system is an important part of your health. Yang practises that include sun salutations and inversions, especially headstands, ensure the movement of the lymphatic system, which is dependent on movement to function.

Words associated with *yang* are solid, movement, warm, active, functional, and creative. A good yang practise also stimulates your sympathetic creative system and releases trapped energy in you. A bad practise will deplete your energy by dipping into your *chi*, the finite core energy with which you are born. When your *chi* runs out, you basically drop dead. In Yoga, I have heard it explained in a different way. You are born with a certain number of breaths. When you finish this finite amount, you are kaput. This makes sense because if your breathing is fast and shallow, you are most likely sitting in stress and fear, and, well, you know the sequence by now.

So Human, if you have been running around all day like a nut case and are exhausted, Yang is not the practise for you. It will deplete you. Now, if you have been sitting around all day, feeling lazy and immobile, then a yang practise is perfect because in these practises you are activating your energetic self.

Yang practises are popular these days in the human world as humans tend to shy away from silence and stillness. They never want to hear themselves because they are afraid of what they will hear. There is the ever-popular *vinyasa*, though few who practise it know what a *vinyasa* is. It is the process by which you flow from up to down, to plank onto your stomach, lifting your chest, and then coming back into down dog."

Orangutan paused for a moment and demonstrated a *vinyasa*. We all applauded as really it was a sight to see.

"A *vinyasa* practise will tie poses together with this flow. It seeks to dump stress, build strength, and increase the circulation of blood and oxygen, especially to places where your muscles are

Asanas Practised by Orangutan

overly contracted. Vinyasa starts to loosen the body, and although it does stretch, its focus is more on strength.

Ashtanga, the physical practise that originated from a system of *hatha*, is a slower style of Yoga. It connects the body's movement with breath and focus. *Iyengar*, like Ashtanga, has its foundation in the eight limbs of Yoga set out by rishi Patanjali, whose Yoga story we are retelling here. An *iyengar* practise focus more on alignment and the use of props to ensure you are structurally correct, and your focus is directed toward a body part. *Kundalini* Yoga fundamentally seeks, through rapid movements and breath, to open and balance your chakras and awaken the *kundalini shakti* in you.

A good Yoga class will focus on traditional Yoga poses as these mirror your bodies energetic systems. They are meant to be repeated, so over time you can slowly bring your body back to its proper alignment and structure, a place where nothing is squashed, twisted, or buried, and all your organs and glands are deeply massaged.

Hatha Yoga, one of the oldest forms of Yoga, is a balance between Yin and Yang Yoga and seeks to bring your body back to homeostasis (balance). It is a slower practise and poses are held for longer periods. Many say that *hatha* and *ashtanga* are the embodiment of Yoga on a mat.

Then there is Yin Yoga for all your connective tissue, your world-famous fascia, and your mind. Yin is where humans hold poses for three or more minutes. On average, it takes two minutes for your muscles to relax and the tension to move to your connective tissues. Once there, cells known as fibroblasts are released at the site. Their primary functions are to strengthen fibrous connective tissue, increase its flexibility, and maintain, improve, and detoxify the lubrication within your joints. Yin ensures that all your fibrous tissues are connected in an organized way. This is especially true of your fascia, within which sits your communication cable network. Your body really is a self-contained spaceship that can either navigate you through space smoothly or completely fall apart, thereby cutting your journey short.

Yin is also deeply important for your bones. Did you know, Corey, that your body is constantly regenerating itself? Skin cells regenerate every two to four weeks, the liver cells every 150 to 500 days, your stomach cells every five days, and your entire bone network every 10 years. Your whole body changes every twelve years such that there is not one cell in you that was there twelve years ago.

This is why people who practise Yoga's eight limbs begin to look younger. They fuel the regeneration of cells through movement, compression, oxygen, and happy emotions. As you age, Yoga *asanas* reduce the rate at which your regenerative processes slow down.

Within all your bones reside cells called osteocytes that comprise 95% of the living cells in an adult bone. At its simplest explanation, osteocytes communicate with osteoblasts, which are responsible for new bone growth, and osteoclasts, which are responsible for breaking down and reabsorbing bones.

In Yin practises when you send compression to your bones, osteocytes signal osteoblasts to create and form new bone. These cells are so smart that they do so in an organized, coherent fashion. When you are inactive, however, and there is no compression, tension, and stress on the bone and your calcium levels are low, osteocytes change allegiances asking osteoclasts to reabsorb nutrients from your bones, thereby weakening them."

In Chinese medicine, Yin also ignites your meridians, or the energy channels that are connected to all your organs. In doing so, it gives your organs a good shaking and boost of energy to ensure that they are working at their optimal level and your emotions remain in balance.

At the level of the mind, unlike yang Yoga that increases your focus, Yin seeks to move you to a place of introspection and to allow the mind to sit in a state of calmness, so it may observe your mind, your *koshas*, conditionings, habits, and addictions from a place of nonattachment. In holding space for silence, Yin also gifts you the time to let go of your attachment to your thoughts and to release them from bondage, thereby allowing you to slowly move to a place of knowing your true self.

Now Human, before we end today, let me give you some tips, so you may begin to dive into the world of *asanas*."

Orangutan began to physically present the words that were dropping from her beautiful, hairy face.

"Always start your practise with five to ten yogic breaths to bring your mind into the present, onto the mat, and into your body and to calm your mind and therefore your breath. Take stock of your body and where you may be holding stress or injuries. Note where you feel heavy and where you feel light and spacious. Be sure to be present throughout your practise. Breathing through the heaviness creates more space within you for light to enter. Set an intention for your practise of a change you want to see in you.

If you have been sitting all day, begin with some sun salutations to warm your body, get oxygen to all your muscles, and remove the stress and carbon dioxide from you. Here are some general rules. Enter forward bends before back bends. Remember that forward bends encourage introspection, a journey inward, as well as cleansing the liver, spleen, and digestive organs among others, whereas back bends open you up to the infinite possibilities that exist out in the Universe for you. They are the place where the impossible is possible. They also work on such areas as your kidney and adrenal glands. In forward bends, shut out the external world. In back bends, shed you labels, your judgement, your stereotypes, step out of your boxes, and just lay yourself open to the Universe and surrender.

Work your core before entering back bends. Always do a twist after a back bend to neutralise the spine. Try and end your practise with an inversion, a headstand or shoulder stand. Inversions boost your immune system. Every muscle has an antagonist, so if you are stretching or strengthening your hamstrings, make sure you also work your quads and psoas muscles. To do one without the other is to risk injury. It is well worth investing in a Yoga anatomy book to better understand your anatomy. Finish with one or two restorative poses and then a *savasana*. Even if the *savasana* is for two minutes, it allows your body to create memory and heal."

"Now Corey, come down here, so I can show you how to do a headstand. Elephant, can you come a little closer to act as a support for Corey should his balance falter?"

Elephant lumbered over and got down onto all fours. Orangutan led Corey to kneel such that the side of Elephant was facing him. At this point, I figured we could ask a whale shark to open its mouth and ask Corey to enter and he would. We all laughed at the thought, except for Corey who was too concentrated on the task at hand to hear any of us.

"Now, get on all fours and place your elbows in-line with your shoulders. Then bend your forearms inward, so there is a hand wrapped around each elbow. What we are doing here is setting up the correct alignment. Now open the forearms, without moving the elbows, and make a cup with your hands. Place the crown of your head on the earth and support the back of your head with the cupped hands. Now slowly, keeping the forearms grounded and pushed into the earth, lift the lower half of you into a downward facing dog pose. Begin to walk your feet toward your hands. When you get to the point where your feet start to lift off the ground, lift one leg and then the other, using Elephant's side to support you."

We watched as Corey kicked his legs up and Orangutan took them and held them up toward the sky. She then gently pushed his legs against Elephant's, who oddly was tickled and giggled. She did this just to show him that there was a support there and he ought not to allow fear to enter him.

"Corey, don't worry. I have got you in the front. Now push your forearms into the earth almost as if you want to lift your head off the earth. The foundation of headstand is all in your arms and shoulders not in your neck. Now, gently squeeze your skeleton, as you do in mountain pose, and push the bush."

"Push what?" Corey exclaimed.

"You know, the bush. That mound between your legs. Push it slightly forward to bring it into alignment."

I could hear upside-down giggles everywhere.

"Tada! You got it, Corey, the king of Yoga poses. Now stay here for five breaths, breathing through the nose and with your eyes open. Balance becomes more challenging with your eyes closed. One day, you will be able to do this without an elephant and with your eyes closed."

When Corey was finished, Orangutan helped him lower his legs and then put him into a child's pose, where he remained to allow all the blood to return to its designated areas. As he slowly rolled his spine up, we could see the glow in him. Headstands are great for bringing you back to happiness.

"Thank you Orangutan and Elephant. That was amazing. I was afraid of that pose and had convinced myself that it was not important. Given the right alignment, it was easier and felt more powerful than I thought."

"You're welcome, Mr. Corey. It is because most people believe that they need to stand on their head, which is painful and uncomfortable to the neck. Try and do one every day, as long as your nose is not blocked, for as long as your arms will hold you. Now I think we are done today, so if you will excuse me, I am going to dance over to a banana."

I turned to the sky. "Thank you, lightning bugs, for lighting our path today. It has bought all of us to a wonderland of possibility. Now, Corey, if it is okay with you, I am going to allow some of the fireflies to escort you back. They are wanting to share their magnificence with you."

His disappointment was palpable, which I understood for it had been some time since I had accompanied him back to duality, but he was not mine to own. It was important that as many of us as possible connected to him. I knew that a time would come when there would be no separation between us. He did not need my physical presence to feel my love or for me to accompany him. I sat in his heart and he in mine.

15

The Magic of Doing Nothing: A Lion's World

We had decided to meet at sunrise today because it was the part of the day we cherished most. It brought with it the hope of a new day, a chance to reset and start again. We knew that there was no such thing as perfection and that all beings faltered, especially humans. Therefore, the rising sun was an opportunity to shed the past and start a new present.

I had asked Corey to come straight to the cove. We, the inhabitants of the cove, were meeting earlier in the hours just before sunrise when silence is at its best and filled with peace and hope of a better day. Each day moves us all closer to a world guided by light not darkness. We met to discuss ways by which each of us could spread the knowledge that was being shared here to the rest of humanity.

We were beginning to understand that humans had to be open and ready for this knowledge. We could not shove it down their throats. We could only love them into Yoga. Through love, they would begin to see the power of what we were teaching. For in darkness, turmoil, war, and chaos, love remains a constant.

Corey arrived just as the sun began to peek at us from across the horizon. It was a ball of fire, shimmering in the heat. It arrived with joy and gratitude, its orange outfit like no other we had seen in nature. And the vibration it came with was AUM. No matter what state you are in, when the rising sun makes its entrance, you move to *sattva*.

We all sat in silence, breathing in unison: five counts in, holding in relaxation for two, ten counts out, holding at the bottom for two. There was a smile breaking out on all our faces that was helping our nostrils to expand to allow for a greater exchange of oxygen and carbon dioxide and the intake of *prana*.

Corey quietly padded barefoot over to Ocean and sat at the edge among us. He settled onto his sitting bones and synchronized his breath with ours. We sat like that until the rising sun was replaced with rays of light breaking through the slits in the clouds. A waterfall of rays across the entire Ocean was singing a song so joyous that it could be heard in our silence. We all heard it, not with our ears but with our souls. It was magnificent how it enveloped all the space and wrapped itself around our hearts. You knew as you sat there that you were listening to the Universe.

We placed our hands over our heart and set an intention for the new day ahead of us, for a change we wanted to see within ourselves. We always preferred our intentions to be a change in us not in our lives. We knew that if we changed, everything would change to reflect us.

Then we did our three deep AUMs, rubbed the palms of our hands, and placed them over our eyes. On the next exhale, we lowered them and opened our eyes as we arrived out of darkness and into light.

"Welcome holders of light and love. I thank you once again for honouring the Human with your presence and knowledge. Take a moment to find a spot in an umbrella to the sun or under the sun as we begin our journey into restorative Yoga and the disco that it plays in our body.

But before we begin, I would like to water a seed we have been planting. Human, you are not the animal that society keeps telling you that you are. You are not selfish, bad, or evil. Your instinct is not to divide, kill, or be alone. The instinct that society tells you rises from your animal brain, we animals can testify are not behaviours from animals. Yes, we engage in death to survive, but take that off the table and we are kind, loving, caring beings. Most of us live in pods, packs, prides, troops, some form of community. Humans too are social beings at your very core. Do not allow anyone to tell you different. When you take this journey of Yoga and connect to your true self, you will reconnect to the love and goodness that is you. When you do, where you once felt lost and untethered, you will now be grounded and see your way clearly."

As we settled in, Corey did his rounds greeting nature and then settled under Willow tree and the shade it afforded his luminous white skin.

"Today, Lion is going to tell us this story for he is well acquainted with doing nothing for nearly 20 hours out of a 24-hour day."

"Ahhh, come on Eagle, you jest. It is not nothing I am doing. I am rejuvenating my form, so it may hunt to feed my family. Hunting is not an easy feat without a gun. Plus, it takes enormous energy to protect my pride, play with my young, and procreate."

"Don't worry, Lion. We are merely teasing you. You are not the only one in the nonhuman kingdom that engages in restorative Yoga every day. We all love it. Humans should learn that doing nothing is so beneficial to their health. Come. Tell the Human this story."

Lion slowly walked over to Corey. Each step created a ripple across all his muscles, and then he sat on his hind legs in front of the Human. It was a sight we would never forget.

"Corey, humans live in this strange world that awards productivity and slanders them for doing nothing. As a result, you all walk around wearing the sheriff's badge of stress. You only feel worthy of this badge if you are constantly running around, being stressed, and doing something productive. You swap the stress badge for the guilt one when you do nothing, and yet it is nothing that will save you in the world in which you live.

Restorative Yoga is a physical practise where you are guided into poses with the use of props to completely relax your body. The practise aims to fill the gaps between you and the Earth such that you feel little or no sensation in your body, and then all the cells and systems in your body have a party: your immune system, your digestive system, well, basically all your systems. They all sing and dance because there is no stress, no stimulation, no drama, nothing to pull it and all its cells away from their job. They engage in some serious disco as they begin to do the jobs they were created to do. They repair, heal, rejuvenate, and, best of all, regenerate all your cells, organs, bones, etc. They fix you, hug you, and revive you, so at the end of a class, you feel calm and energetic. This is because you release energy that has been kidnapped by stress and your muscles. It does not matter what age you are, by embracing the discipline of Yoga, you can begin to reverse illnesses, diseases, turn off harmful genes, and regenerate your inner self for a healthier inner and outer self. Yoga is magic because it works from the inside out.

Too many humans believe that changing the outside will change them inside. All the alterations you constantly make to your hair, face, and body with makeup, clothes, hair products, etc., change nothing on the inside. No, wait. I am lying to you here. It does change the inside; it keeps you in such low-frequency emotions as insecurity and all those other unhealthy emotions that rise with the attachment to anything external and impermanent.

Restorative Yoga is so powerful because it teaches your body to relax, thereby creating new memories, habits, and reactions to emotions and stressors stored in your amygdala, which is your emotional storage unit, so the next time you are stressed, you seek relaxation and calmness instead of anger, anxiety, booze, weed, etc. You know, Human, restorative Yoga is just a journey into *savasana*. *Savasana* is one of the most challenging poses for humans as you struggle to completely relax and surrender without the aid of anything but your breath.

It is also a practise that allows for the creation of a safe space in which you can observe your thoughts and emotions from a point of objectivity and not feel powerless to do anything about them. When you have trauma sitting in you, it is the feeling of being unsafe and powerless that allows your traumas to block you from moving forward. A good restorative Yoga practise creates a safe space where you feel in control to observe your conditionings, your experiences, and your thoughts, without them triggering you, so you can begin to dismantle them and release them.

Restorative poses also allow for your nervous system to reset and bring your body back into homeostasis, which at the same time activates your body's healing system. Most humans, Corey, are either living with their sympathetic system dominating, meaning you are always reacting to things and are constantly engaged in your senses, or with their parasympathetic system dominating, meaning you spend an inordinate amount of time sleeping, inactive, or in a sloth-like slumber.

Both result in feeling a complete lack of control over your life and your emotions, as well as a weakened immune and digestive systems among other things. This manifests on the outside as dry skin, hair loss, rashes, etc. Restorative Yoga, *savasana*, Yoga *nidra*, and traditional Yoga practises are so important because they all seek to bring you back into homeostasis.

What you want is for the parasympathetic nervous system to be in balance and healthy such that its star player, the vagus nerve, can efficiently play the whole field that is your body. The wandering tenth cranial nerve is the only cranial nerve to leave the brain and go for a walk throughout the body. Its arms and legs extend into every major organ in your body like a caterpillar, acting as the informant that communicates between the organs and the brain. One of the most important of these links is to your gut, home to more immune cells than anywhere else in our body.

The vagus nerve originates in the brain stem and runs down the human throat. Therefore, beginning any practise with chanting a mantra creates a vibration that will stimulate the nerve. AUM is particularly powerful as it allows your diaphragm to contract at length, thereby squeezing the vagus nerve that, along with your oesophagus, runs through your diaphragm. When this happens, it releases a substance known as oxyacetylene. This substance slows down your heartbeat and reduces inflammation in the body. AUM also initiates a vibration in your throat, the other place where you stimulate and massage your vagus nerve, through the long M at the end of the AUM.

By the way, gargling warm salt water after every tooth brushing also massages and stimulates your vagus nerve as well as the killing any bacteria hanging around at the back of your throat.

Now Corey, what I am trying to explain to you is important because the vagus nerve is the most important component of the parasympathetic system and plays a multitude of roles, including creating new brain neurons, repairing brain tissue, and exciting stems cells to create new cells. More importantly, a healthy vagus nerve prevents inflammation in the gut from bypassing the blood brain barrier and using a weakened vagus nerve to cause inflammation in the brain.

But what I really want to speak about today is the relationship between the vagus nerve and the heart and why it is so important to balance your nervous systems with such practises as Yin and restorative.

Now, stay with me because I am going to try and simplify this. Remember your brain stem? Where all your autonomic systems that you can influence but have no control over reside? Well, two of the autonomic systems that carry on whether you are consciously present or not are your respiratory system, which sits in your brain stem, and your circulatory system. Which, by the way, is the same for all of us beings."

Lion stopped and pondered for a minute on how best to explain how this all worked. It was important for humans to have knowledge of how their own systems worked. They kept ingesting things without any awareness of what went on in their systems, their mind, their energy, and inevitably their consciousness.

"Okay, I think I have it. Human, close your eyes and follow the visual I am about to create for you. Which I can do because my sympathetic system, the home of my unique creativity, is very much in balance.

Visualise your respiratory system as housed in a magical temple inside your brain stem. In this temple, there are numerous happy tiny breathing gurus sitting around a large table getting high on oxygen. In this same temple lives a long, beautiful two-legged yellow caterpillar called vagus. Now, visualise one of its legs, the left one, extending out of the temple directly to the heart, where it attaches to the SA node that sits on the top part of the heart the atrium. Its right leg extends out and connects to the AV node on the heart that controls the expansion and contraction of the ventricles.

The SA node is responsible for setting the rhythm of the heart; it is the pacemaker. When triggered, it contracts the top part of your heart and a sends an electrical signal to the AV node to expand and then contract the lower part of the heart. The right part is responsible for sending blood to your lungs and the left to the rest of your body.

Now, also in the temple is a bright blue snake connected to your sympathetic nervous system. That snake slithers out of the temple and runs down your spine to where it offshoots into a gang of smaller fibre snakes that connects to the SA node on the pacemaker part of the heart.

In addition to the stoned gurus, the caterpillar, and the snake, there are friends of the gurus, known as *sufis*. These *sufis* sit in other parts of the body and report to the gurus any shifts that require a change in heartbeat. For example, in the blood stream these *sufis* are known as chemoreceptors that monitor oxygen and carbon dioxide levels in the blood. In the lungs, the *sufis* are known as mechano-receptors that monitor the stretch in the lung muscles. Believe it or not, there is such a thing as stretching the lung muscles too much. Then there are other *sufis* in the hypothalamus that monitor hormonal changes due to stress. Others hang out in your frontal cortex, where they seek to consciously influence your breath and, therefore, your heart rate.

These *sufis* are in constant communication with the gurus and sending them messages on the state of all the systems. The gurus then use the information to determine your heart rate and rhythm or to tell the heart to just stop. You see, the gurus are a peaceful sort, and, at some point, if they can´t keep up with the overload of negative information that the *sufis* keep sending them, they will seek peace and balance and just stop the heart.

When you practise restorative Yoga, you slow down your breath, so there is an optional exchange of oxygen and carbon dioxide. As your breath slows down, so do your thoughts, sending a signal to your hypothalamus that all is good. When all is well, there is no need to increase cortisol levels or dump harmful chemicals in you. As a result, your body calms down and enters a safe and secure zone such that no extra blood needs to be pumped to your extremities. The *sufis* signal the gurus that all is calm, who in turn signal the yellow parasympathetic caterpillar to slow down the heart by slowing the electrical pulses in the SA and AV nodes. At the same time, it puts the blue sympathetic snake on a leash. In doing so, it asks your body to basically move out of a fast-paced sympathetic flamingo dance and into a rhythmic, calm, slow parasympathetic dance.

And while the heart slow dances, the rest of your systems kicks into disco as they start to heal wounds, kill cells plagued by diseases, regenerate dying cells, open blocked energy centres, and bring you to a place of awareness. The latter allows you to then retreat from the external world and enter your internal world.

The Magic of Doing Nothing

Humans, your body is miraculous!

Yoga teaches your body to move into this state right after a stressful event, or even before a stressful event. When you can do this, you are freeing your self from antibiotics, vaccines, illnesses, and diseases. A body that is in homeostasis will bounce back from a stressful event within a very short period instead of continuing to sit in the stress of the event long after the event has passed.

But how do you know how well you are doing, especially if your connection to yourself is somewhat dodgy? Well, there is a human gadget that can help you: a HRV ring.

HRV stands for heart rate variability, which is the space between heartbeats. A shorter time between heart beats indicates that your body is sitting in your sympathetic flight-or-fight flamingo dance system. As the space between heart beats lengthens, your body begins to move back into balance, and your parasympathetic slow dance system is activated.

When playing with an HRV ring, there are two things you want to track. One is how long after you have been in a stressful event it takes for the space between heartbeats to get longer. In other words, the recovery rate of your body from imbalance to balance. The other is to check your HRV when you are feeling fine and calm. If in this state your HRV is still low, meaning that the space between your heartbeats is short, then there is something going on inside of you that should not be going on. It's like having a straight guy at a disco purely for gays. Not easy to spot, blends in okay, so you think all is normal, but he should not be there.

Corey, please understand that everything humans need to heal yourselves, to be a healthy sane human not afflicted by diseases, mental illness, and depression, exits within them. In fact, you have an entire pharmacy inside of you. You can produce in your body most of those drugs you buy to make you feel better or get you high. Yes, even ayahuasca.

We in the rest of nature are always surprised at how humans work so hard for cars, homes, clothes, and security, but when asked to do that same work on yourselves, to do nothing, to eat well, come to your mats, meditate, etc., you just keep opting out and claiming you don't have the time. By doing this, you keep riding that blue snake until one day you drop dead from something that was preventable had you done the work.

There you have it, Corey, a journey into the human form and a deeper understanding of why so many of us in the animal kingdom recline ourselves into rest for such long periods. Though mind you, we are not as bad as the bear that hibernates for months. Anyway, the reason we do it and you don't is not because we are lazy, it's because we are geniuses."

The cove erupted into uncontrollable laughter at the compliment Lion had paid them.

"In ending, let me add a little homework for you. To know what is going on inside of you, it is not enough to just observe your body when you are on the mat. Begin to observe your tongue, your poop, your skin, your hair, your nails, and so forth off the mat. They are all manifestations of what is going on inside of you. Rashes, dry skin, brittle hair, constipation, discoloured faeces, and white tongue are just some of the warning signs that your body is not in homeostasis, and all is not well with you.

Give thanks to water and food before it enters you because positive energy affects the chemical and cellular composition of all elements. When you go to the toilet to poo, place your legs on a stool, close your eyes, and in silence visualise all the toxins slowly moving through you and then out of you. Clean your colon, and when you are done, thank your body. Don't sit on a phone or read a book. Be present in every act that you perform. Trust me: your body, mind, and soul will thank you for it."

"Wow. That was great. Thank you, Lion. The whole thing has made me wonder about reincarnation and the belief Yogis have that the human is the ultimate form for consciousness to reside in before being liberated. Because from where I sit, you animals seem to have it right." Corey paced around. His mind was sparking all over the place.

"I agree, Corey. It is the one place where we divert from the yogic discipline. But we shall get into that another day. It is hot, and many of us would like to enter a restorative pose to conserve our energy for the much-needed hunt to feed ourselves. You are welcome to slumber with us if you do not need to rush off to some task."

"You know what? I think I will stay. I am beginning to understand that sitting on a couch and watching a screen is not, in fact, restorative to my body at all. It is going to be hard, but I am going to have to learn to rest, not sleep, without stimulation or the company of anything but my breath."

I sighed in joy. He was important to me, to all of us, and we wanted nothing but the best for him even if it meant that maybe one day we would have to let him go. It was a thought I did not want to give energy to, so I did not. As I shook myself out of the well of thoughts into which I had dived, I found myself amid a siesta on the grandest scale. My vision found Corey under a tree. His head was on Leopard, Snake at his feet, and Orangutan hanging over his head. I flew over and perched beside him. I placed my wing on his chest and closed my eyes. In the silence, I could hear all of life in the hundreds of inhales and exhales that mingled with the space in which it lived. It was a breath that was *sattvic* in nature. There was no rush, no negativity, just peace. It was how it was meant to be.

16

Prana, The Forgotten One

I felt my breath as I perched on the limb of the highest tree overlooking the cove. I noticed it was shallow, short, and erratic, erupting from my chest. It was reflecting the unease that was flowing back and forth within me, like the tide of Ocean. I knew that to stop it all I had to do was lengthen my exhales, slow down my heartbeat, and pull my mind back into the present.

But instead, I sat in my unease, without attachment, and observed what it was telling me. Humans spend an inordinate amount of time running away from pain, burying it in places to one day come back to haunt them at a higher volume. Our pain is constantly highlighting our attachments and guiding us to learn the lesson that come with every sorrow. Little do humans understand that pain comes for a reason, to cleanse, to teach, to give rise to awareness, and to heal. To be human is to endure and experience suffering; it is the way their form is set up.

I knew the Human was struggling, and my heart bled for him. As we entered the last part of the love story between the self and the Universe, I knew that much would rise to the surface for him. And when it did, I knew all too well that there was a chance he would shut himself down and walk away from me and the cove. My unease was telling me that we would need to tread slowly and gently here and to be supportive, no matter what came to the surface. My unease was also telling me to let go of my attachment to him. It had happened so slowly and unconsciously that I had not been aware of it.

As I flapped my wings with all my strength, I gave space and an avenue for my feelings to move out of me instead of burying them into my bones and my feathers. I landed on a large rock that was elevated on one end and flattened into a natural seat on the other. From there, I watched Corey walk down the path toward me. His wide chest and solid legs strode forward with purpose, as if he were on his way to conquer the world.

When he saw me, his face expanded as his smile pushed itself outward. "Eagle, what a pleasant surprise. It has been a long time since you met me at this place where we become one."

"Hello Corey, yes it has. We in the rest of nature are not used to speaking so much. It is an energy drainer, so I find my naps have got a little longer."

"Naps, I can't remember the last time I had a nap. I think I was three. Though after the restorative story, I have started engaging in some poses every evening, instead of comatosing myself with TV. Now, to what do I owe this pleasure?"

"Here, come sit beside me."

"Ahhh, the sitting beside you action, should I be scared?"

"Hahahaha, no, not at all. We are moving into energy and breath, and then into meditation. All tools to heal, to help move you to self-love, and to reconnect you with your true self. But to create any lasting shift in you, to give rise to change, there must be four things in place. The first is awareness of the conditioned self and all that it is giving rise to in you. The second is acceptance of all that you witness. The third is to let go of all that does not serve you well, and the fourth is to surrender to the Universe that exists within you and trust that it will guide you in the right direction.

"Today we will continue to lay the foundation for the above to happen as we move into *prana* and breath. When you return to your human heavy world, we ask that you begin to do the following:

Begin everyday with sitting in silence for 15 minutes. While following your breath, begin to be aware of the habitual thoughts your mind keeps ruminating on. Make note of your mental habits and then come back to your breath. Try and listen to what appears before you in the silence between each breath.

Then as you move through each day, start to practise your *yamas* and *niyamas*. To do so, you will have to be aware of all your thoughts, actions, and behaviors when you are on your own and when you interact with others. Because to practise them, to know that you are following them, you must be aware of your mind. Take a note of where you falter, where you struggle to adhere to them, and ask yourself why. Every answer must come from a place of truth. To access your truth, you must shed any judgements of yourself, disengage from fear, and accept what you hear.

Do not worry. As we have already told you, in the beginning you will fail at mastering the *yamas* and *niyamas*, but through the process of sticking with them, it will become easier and easier as you cleanse the mind. The beginning will be a battle. The mind will always seek to find ways to justify and make an excuse for an exception to a *yama* or *niyama*. But trust us, to enact lasting change you must follow them. And when you fail to do so, you must seek the answers within as to why you failed. For these are your guides to knowing you.

This journey we are asking you to embark on requires you to dedicate time to you to move from a reactive state to a responsive state. Change takes time and effort. Corey, you will have to make the time every day to sit in silence and do nothing but observe and listen.

It is time for you to get off the fence. To choose a side, either the involution toward your true self or to remain in the comfort of the victim. You must seek help when you are unsure to not interpret knowledge in a way that suits you or justifies actions that are not good for you or all living beings. You know, Corey, knowledge is very dangerous in the hands of those who do not fully understand it. We animals sometimes speak of how the printing press of ancient scriptures was what has given rise to so many wars around religion. Because any man who can read, can now take correct knowledge and disperse it incorrectly to the masses. You know, there was a reason knowledge was given orally and transferred only to those who were ready for it."

I looked over at Corey, and in silence, he nodded. "I will try my best. I may have to quit my job to find the time for me and throw my TV and phone out the window, but I will find the time. But before we go, I wanted to ask you about psychedelics. In my world, there is a lot of talk these days about the benefits of them in enacting healing and removing the ego."

"Ah yes. I shall not say much about this except that there is great value in them for those seeking to move through trauma and know that there exists something larger than all of us. It is a tool used by medicine men and spiritual thinkers to connect and gain knowledge. They are powerful in forcing you to acknowledge the small ego in you that keeps you attached to everything outside of you. But true change takes work. The eradication of fear, the ability to change your reality, the courage to shed your life of materialism, all takes work. Psychedelics are not a fast fix or to be taken constantly. They are incredible tools to bring about awareness of the Universe and to flame the fuel of *tapas*, self-knowledge.

Over time, this has eroded humans' belief and awareness that there is something larger than all of you. As humans have become more disillusioned by religion, they have turned to capitalism, power, and money as their belief system. As a result, your species has crumbled because as far as they are concerned, this is it. They live in their desires and do everything in excess and suffer. Your world increasingly looks like constant chaos, with nearly eight billion people living in their desires. There is an enormous need for Yoga in your human world, and we ask nothing of you but to take the time, do the work, and let the rest fall into place. Come, let us wander to the cove."

I flew onto Corey's shoulder, and we began the walk. The silence between us was beautiful and had grown as the distance between us had diminished.

When we arrived at the cove, we found all of nature in a restorative pose. We could feel the healing and at the same time the rejuvenation of life all around us. Warm rain began to fall from Sky, giving birth to new life and sustaining existing life. With each step, Corey felt Earth sing below his bare feet and the trees sway as they feasted on the gift that enveloped them. Water, how humans in the West took it for granted. They believe that water, like everything, including breath, is infinite.

All the beings rolled into an upright position as we entered the cove. In one large *namaste* they greeted us, smiling through the gentle patter of rain. I placed Corey under the protection of a tree, and I flew over Ocean to take a moment to immerse myself in the joy that was being played out below me. The marine world sang, jumped, flipped, and dove, each one grateful for their world and all that inhabited it.

As I landed back on the tree, the rain stopped and a rainbow appeared. It was a magnificent piece of art that refracted all the frequencies of the Universe's white light, a reminder that at the root of all diversity there is unity. We all came from the same place, and although our journeys are different, we all seek the same destination.

"Namaste nature, it is good to see all of you washed clean of your impurities and glistening as if reborn. Today we will begin the journey into breath and *prana*. You know, that thing humans don't really pay attention to? Humans are such a funny species. They keep seeking ways to cheat death, but the one thing that determines whether they live or die in this form, they ignore: breath. I have asked one of the whales to tell you this story today because they have a breath that is similar humans'."

As I ended my last words, I heard Whale break through the surface and begin a slow swim across the cove. We all watched as she stretched in leaps and bounds, her young beside her, until finally she settled into a slow glide. We, in turn, settled into our selves, turned the volume of our minds down, and connected to her frequency.

"Hello beings. We have listened much and spoken little, absorbing all the knowledge being shared here. Just as we have listened from our soul, it is from my soul that I shall speak today.

We have spoken much about stilling the mind. However, there is another path within you to calm the mind, and that path is through your breath. When your breath is calm and constant, your mind is more peaceful and observation becomes much easier. As you can imagine, it is so much harder to move to a place of self-awareness and observation if your breath is in the middle of a bullfight.

In Yoga, breath is the vehicle that carries *prana* throughout your body and the conduit between your mind and body. *Prana* is energy that pervades your entire being and is present everywhere in nature. However, humans struggle to absorb it from nature due to the resistance in your breath from incorrect breathing techniques. Humans, like the rest of us, absorb *prana* from all the energetic elements within which all life exists.

For example, Earth's energy can be absorbed through eating fresh fruits and veggies, walking barefoot on Earth, and by just being in nature. To absorb energy from the water element, drink plenty of pure water devoid of chemicals. To gain *prana* from fire, visit Sun, drink warm water, and eat warm foods cooked over a flame. However, the main source of *prana* for humans is breathing. The inhalation of fresh air, airing out the rooms you live and work in, and staying away from polluted environments. Lastly, there is the ether element, which is associated with thoughts. By chanting mantras, keeping positive company, and being in a healthy atmosphere, you can increase your *prana* through the thinking of and listening to positive thoughts.

As you are starting to see, Corey, *prana* is an actor, not a thinker, and is more than just your respiratory process. The process of inhalation, exhalation, and retention are merely indicators that *prana* is alive and working within you. You can't see prana or touch it, but for sure you can feel it. It is like a chicken and egg. It is the *prana* in you that takes in air and expels it from you, and it is that process of inhalation and exhalation that indicates that you have *prana*. One does not exist without the other.

Pranayama is the process through which you can control your breath and by extension your energy. It controls how much you absorb and its distribution into five different areas in the human body, known as *vayus*.

If you can learn to control these five *vayus* through various *pranayamas*, your human form will be devoid of ailments and diseases. Each *vayu* contributes to balancing you mentally as well as physically by keeping you in a *sattvic* state. When you are in a *rajasic* or *tamasic* state, you will struggle to absorb *prana*. However, before I explain the five *vayus*, allow me to give you a better understanding of the three states we keep referring to, known collectively as the *gunas*.

Humans are always moving between three states, known as *gunas*. The first is *sattva*, your purest state where you act out of knowledge, sit in contentment, joy, positivity, and gratitude. In this state you are liberated from violence, fear, and malice. The second is *rajasic*, where you are in a state of action and movement, which manifests in attachment and a longing for the satisfaction of your desires. The last is *tamas*. In this state, you are envcloped by darkness, negativity, anger, jealousy, and all other destructive emotions. *Gunas* are present in everything, even food. There are foods that make you lazy, foods that make you feel good, and foods that incite anger.

Now back to the five Vayus and *prana*. The fundamental essence of *prana* is activity (*rajasic*). It is prana that drives all your systems, so it can never really take a nap. If it does, then rest assured you are dead. Did you know that death is actually the process of *prana* leaving your body? Because, you will remember, *prana* is the energy upon which your consciousness rides.

When you are alive, *prana* uses breath as the vehicle to move it around the body. When the breath is calm and controlled, *prana* is able to move freely around the body. Therefore, *pranayamas* are breathing techniques to keep the vehicle of breath in shape and well maintained. Just imagine how many areas of your body are devoid of energy when your breath is shallow and scattered.

Prana, The Forgotten One

When *prana* enters the body and the breath is flowing freely, it splits into five *vayus*, known as *pancha prana*. Each *vayu* is responsible for taking care of certain operations in the body. The first is *prana*, the inhale, whose job it is to obtain energy from the five elements external to the body and absorb it into the body. The location of this system is in the chest below the neck, so the thoracic and diaphragmic area. It is predominantly responsible for the respiratory and cardiovascular systems (heart, lung, breathing, swallowing, blood circulation), and its energy system moves upward.

On an emotional level, it is responsible for your emotions absorbing information and controlling the mind. Most chest or respiratory diseases can be healed by the *prana vayu*. Aliments that highlight an imbalance in this *vayu* are colds, flus, bronchitis, and a disorientation of the mind. *Pranayamas* with strong inhales keep you mentally strong and emotionally stable. To aid this system, there are also such yoga *asanas* as chest openers, back bends, warrior three, and lunges.

Upon death, the leaving of *prana* is seen by the stopping of the heart, and a loss of the energetic pranic shield which yogis say extends twelve inches from the body. Ever notice how when you are strong and healthy, your energy extends outside of you, but when you are weak, your whole outer self seems to shrink? You can immediately sense if someone is sick or well when you first meet them, without even asking them. You feel it in the energy that surrounds them or lack thereof.

The second *vayu* is the *samana vayu*, which is located between the diaphragm and the navel. Its energy moves in a circular motion. Prana in this system generates heat. So when you die, it is the leaving of this energy system from your form that creates a coldness in the corpse. When this system is balanced, it ensures efficient absorption of energy from food and sustains your essence. On a mental and emotional level, it helps you absorb the learning in every experience you have, while letting go of the actual impression.

For example, if you experience something negative, a healthy *samana vayu* helps you learn from that experience, but not hold onto the experience. This ensures that the negative impressions created by the experience do not have the power to influence you in the future. You know you are holding onto the negative impression when you experience bloating, indigestion, and the constant regurgitation of experiences. When it is in balance, you feel healthy all the way to the cellular level.

Asanas that assist *samana* are twists, core work, and forward folded bends. The types of breath that support this system, are *nauli* gut cleansing and *kabal bathi pranayamas*.

Then there is *apana*, the exhaled breath, located below the navel, embracing the reproductive and excretory systems. Its energetic movement is downward. *Apana* is responsible for removing waste and toxins from a human in a number of ways which include pee, faeces, and periods. Therefore, when it is under active, it creates constipation, light periods, and spotting, and when it is overactive, it creates diarrhea and heavy periods. Unbalanced *apana* can also lead to reproductive problems.

On a mental level, *apana* removes unwanted thoughts and negativity. Some *asanas* that support a healthy *apana* are lower ab work, happy baby, child's pose, seated twists, and *halasana*. As for the breath, the best one is *nauli* breath with engaged *bandas*.

The fourth *vayu* is *vyana* which circulates around the entire human form. It distributes the energy from *samana* and *prana* to the entire circulatory system and influences muscle and joint movements. Its energy flows in an outward, circular motion. When imbalanced, you will feel lazy on a mental as well as physical level. You are also more prone to arthritis, joint, and skeletal problems.

However, when in balance, energy flows freely through the body and the mind can flow without resistance. Your body and mind feel lighter as you find you can express yourself more openly. When you die, this energy system takes the longest to leave. It is the process of the body rotting, which is why in some cultures, the body is cremated. To allow a body to rot slowly results in all your energy being released over a longer period of time. There is a belief in cultures that cremate that the soul is not completely released until all the energy, which is also present in every cell, is set free.

The last *vayu* is *udana,* located in the neck and upward. Its energy flows upward, and this system is deeply connected to reasoning, intuition, the neurological system, and analysis. Some call this system the CEO of the body, and it is through this system that humans move to higher states of consciousness. When it is imbalanced, it manifests as depression, loss of cognitive skills, migraines, thyroid issues, and nervous system disorders.

When it is balanced through breath, meditation, and concentration, a human has strong communication skills, thinks clearer, has more awareness, and can even levitate. When the human form dies, this system which is responsible for buoyancy, sinks the body into heaviness.

Asanas to aid this system are shoulder stand, fish, bridge, plow, and headstands. As well as honeybee and *alunoma vilimona* breath, also known as alternate nostril breath.

To practise the limbs of Yoga that are *asanas*, singular focus, and meditation, *prana* needs to flow smoothly and gently through all these systems. For this to happen, you need to be in a *sattvic* state. And we are back to the chicken and the egg because to get into a *sattvic* state, your energy must be flowing smoothly and for your energy to flow smoothly you must be in a *sattvic* state.

But fear not: there is a starting point for the uninterrupted flow of energy, which we shall get into at our next lesson. I think it is enough for today, do you not think so, Eagle?"

"I completely agree. Come, Corey, and let me walk you out today." We both turned to Whale and bowed deeply. "Whale, thank you for your time and knowledge today. You are a master orator."

Whale bowed back and showed her pleasure by creating a fountain from her blowhole. We laughed out loud as the warm water washed over us, and then she disappeared into the belly of Ocean.

Corey jumped to his feet, pleased to have my company on the way in and out. He turned to the cove and Ocean, bent forward in reverence, and offered his gratitude to each and everyone of those whose energy lifted and sustained him.

We walked in silence, well, he walked and I sat on his shoulder, enjoying the tranquility that had grown between us.

"I love you." Corey stopped and turned to me.

I fell off his shoulder and froze as he kept walking. I had waited long and patiently to hear those words from him and said without resistance and hesitancy. I had never doubted they would arrive for I knew the power of loving someone completely just the way they were. As he turned around to pick me up, he lifted me onto his arm and continued.

"I have felt this opening in me and from it swells this love that I have never experienced before. I have been practising visualisation meditation and changing my neural highways by sitting in the future I seek. And you were right. Sometimes when I am moving through my day, I am overcome by feelings of joy and happiness. The source of which is myself because that happiness is attached to nothing. When that love spreads across my being, all I want to do is share it with others, more specifically you."

I was speechless. A human, in love with me, an Eagle? Wonders never ceased to appear in this world. I watched his blush spread and knew that it had taken an enormous amount of courage for him to speak openly, about his feelings.

"I love you as well. And I know it is not that romantic love humans keep playing with, the foundation of which lies in desires. It is something more pure and beautiful. It is okay to love me, Corey, to surrender to what you are feeling. That love will not hurt you because a love like that holds no fear, lives in the moment, and comes from you. But more importantly, it will always attract a love and frequency that matches yours."

We stopped at the point where his world separated him from me. For a moment we just stood there, me on a rock, him on his feet and just watched the other. We were observing how day by day, our forms were dissolving and what filled that void was a beautiful dance between our energies.

17

How Breath Works: The Trees Speak

I arrived later than usual on account of being stuck in a mating ritual to ensure our survival. I was almost sure Corey would not mind because really, although love crossed all boundaries, procreation did not. They had already started today's lesson as I landed on Baobab´s highest limbs.

I waited a few minutes for I knew it would take Corey some time to find me even as I knew he had already felt me. When he finally did, I watched his face explode into happiness, matching that of my heart. He was the most beautiful human man that I have ever laid eyes on. There was a light in him that was so powerful that on those rare occasions when it had broken through the surface, I had been left standing in amazement. He was a powerful human, who had the gift of light. If he followed the path we had set out for him, he would one day connect with it and begin to live his true purpose.

I tilted my head and began to listen into what Willow Tree was telling Corey. Of course it was right that the trees told this story. They are, after all, in a symbiotic relationship with humans. The tree could live without the humans, but could the human live without trees?

"*Prana* is fundamentally *rajasic* in its nature because, you will remember, if it stops, you die. If that *rajasic* state is fueled by your *tamasic* state of negativity, then your *prana*, which is also influenced by your thoughts and emotional state, will get blocked. This will leave you feeling heavy, prone to sickness, and low in energy. When this happens all your vayus will be weakened.

But when your *prana* is calm and consistently shifting gently from *rajasic* to *sattvic*, then everything works as it should, harmoniously.

How Breath Works: The Trees Speak

This is where *pranayama* enters our story. These breathing techniques used by Yogis subdue, settle, and influence *prana*, so t it may assist you to achieve the goal of Yoga. Slow the mind, slow the *prana*. Slow your *prana*, slow your mind, slow everything, move your body back into homeostasis, and bring disco back into your body. Human, it is such an intertwined system between your body, mind, and consciousness. So much so that to really incur change and gain the full benefits of Yoga, it is not enough to engage in just one limb of Yoga. You must slowly and eventually engage in all eight limbs to ensure that your *sattvic guna* is the one that rises to the top of your being, sinking the other two.

If when you first start Yoga, slow *asana* practises and meditation seem like a torture chamber trying to kill you, it is mostly likely because your *rajasic* and *tamas gunas* are in dominance. It is for this same reason, that most of humans struggle with long deep inhales and exhales originating from the diaphragm. Unless you are calm or have experience with *pranayama*, trying to corral your breath is like trying to tame a bull in a bullfight.

So, what is the breath we engage in when practising all aspects of Yoga? Because if you practise Yoga, you will know there are so many different types of breathing, depending on what it is you seek to achieve. There is breath to cool you, to heat you, to vibrate your vagus nerve, to balance your nervous system, and so forth.

For example, when you engage in honeybee breath, you are stimulating the glands in your throat and head, as well as massaging your vagus nerve. When you do *bhastrika* breath, you create heat in your body and a quick release of energy. Then there are cleansing techniques known as *kriyas* that clean and rejuvenate your systems. One such *kriya* is *nauli* breath which decontaminates your digestive system and massages your digestive organs as well as those around them.

But for meditation, which is at the top of the Yoga ladder, only one *pranayama* is required. It is the yogic breath of deep inhales that expand the belly by parachuting open your diaphragm, followed by the rise and expansion of your chest, throat, and the nostrils, without moving the shoulders. Then exhaling deeply without force to completely empty the lungs. In time, your exhale should be much longer than your inhale as you ease your body and mind deeper and deeper into tranquility. Which you will remember from a former class happens on your exhale as it is there that your parasympathetic system's vagus nerve interacts with the breath and then speaks to the heart.

This why so many who sit in anxiety feel a deep pain in their solar plexus as well as feelings of being stuck and heavy. It is because their breath is originating from the chest and not from the belly. As a result, your gut area, the home of your emotions, is unable to move your emotions upward and outward and results in a blockage in both your breath and emotions.

Now Corey, Dragon Tree over there is going to explain the fundamentals of breath to you, so you may have a better idea of how to keep yourself alive without a hospital or a pharmacy."

Just then Dragon Tree stretched his limbs, lengthened his trunk, and took up the baton of breath.

"Hello Corey," he began with his deep, rumbling voice. "Within every human there is a set of nerves called the phrenic nerve that originates from cervical spine three-to-five. Its role is to connect the central nervous system with the diaphragm and to control the expansion and contraction of the diaphragm. These nerves are also responsible for sensory information. They connect the pericardium lining of the heart, the diaphragm, and parts off the lining of the lung together. Therefore, when an injury occurs in one of these regions, pain is can often be felt in one of other regions.

When one or both of these nerves are injured, the diaphragm can no longer contract, and a human is left short of breath. What normally accompanies shortness of breath is anxiety and

How Breath Works: The Trees Speak

fatigue. Let me break it down for you. When you are stressed, you hunch your shoulders and contract your muscles. This places pressure on the neck, which you add to by always looking down at your phone or computer. Rounded shoulders and a compressed neck inhibit your phrenic nerves and block the expansion of your diaphragm. As you move deeper into fatigue and anxiety, you begin to walk hunched over, wanting to hide from the world, for fear of judgment or for fear that others may see how much you are suffering. This posture further blocks your energy and breath, spiralling you further into anxiety.

All of this is aided by a great reduction in the intake of oxygen and *prana* and the dispelling of carbon dioxide. This, Corey, is just another reason Yoga *asanas* for the spine, in fact the whole body, are so important. Proper alignment of your body and movement of *prana* with breath is an integral part of the foundation of Yoga.

The whole breathing structure is made up of so many parts. To begin with, there is the lung, attached to the ribs with a fluid membrane that allows for the smooth movement between the lungs and the ribs with each inhale and exhale. Then there are the core muscles and the muscles around the neck. The muscles around the neck, especially the sternocleidomastoid, lift the sternum to create space for the lungs to expand upward and outward. Other actors that create expansion in the belly and lungs on the inhale are the scalene, which move the ribs, pec minor, which sit to the front of the upper chest, and the diaphragm, of course.

When you inhale, you create a lower pressure cavity in the lung area compared to outside the body. It is this pressure differential that encourages air to flow inwards. Furthermore on the inhale, the diaphragm moves down, creating pressure in the abdominal area to drain blood into the heart and respiratory areas as well as massage all the organs in that area. On the exhale, the core muscles, mostly the obliques and transverse abdominus muscles, pull the rib cage and, by extension, the diaphragm back into place, while squeezing the vegus nerve that runs through it.

Therefore, we encourage you to do a slight contraction of the core muscles at the end of the exhale.

In addition to all the moving parts, there is the entire respiratory centre located in the medulla oblongata, the part of the brainstem that controls your breathing known as the dorsal respiratory group. From this centre, signals are sent to C3, 4, and 5 to speak with the phrenic nerve that contracts the diaphragm.

At the same time, the ventral respiratory system, which is part of the dorsal system, sends signals to all the aforementioned muscles to create contraction and relaxation for the inhale and the exhale. Looking at it from the top down, it looks a little like this: You consciously engage the cerebral cortex to begin to influence your breath. It, in turn, sends a signal to the hypothalamus, which then signals the respiratory centres in the medulla.

If all is well in you, and your shoulders are away from your ears, your chest is open, and your spine aligned, your natural breath will begin from your belly. When you begin to ask your breath to move into your yogi breath, you will begin to influence *prana* to move out of its *rajasic* nature and into its *sattvic*, less stimulated state. As the breath begins to slow down even further, you will be able to slow your thoughts and begin to remove any attachments to your thoughts. Remember that thoughts have the power to catapult your *prana* back to its erratic state.

If you are sitting in a state of constant stress, negative emotions, and your body is misaligned, this whole process is going to be much more challenging. Not impossible, but for sure more of a challenge. You will almost have to reteach yourself how to breathe properly in addition to strengthening parts of your lung muscles that have rarely been used.

Many *pranayamas* should not be done when you are hungry, angry, or in a state of emotional turbulence because if you do, you are right back in the bullfight. In the above states of negativity, one should slowly engage in deep yogic breaths at a lower count, maybe a count of 4 in and 4 out, to allow your mind to shift out of turbulence and into calmness. There should

How Breath Works: The Trees Speak

be no retention of breath to start with. *Prana* must accept the conditions that are going to be imposed on it. Also, when you engage in this yogic breath, it should be mild without sound and unaffected by emotions. As the mind slows, the count can increase.

Eventually when you move to a place where you are on close terms with your energy and your mind is amicable to the practice, you can then engage in the retention of breath on the top of the inhale, bottom of the exhale, or both. However, that retention should never feel like you are suffocating, straining, or creating pain. In fact it should always be retained in your head or solar plexus with relaxation. Both are areas where humans store *prana*.

Only after some time can you then move to alternate nostril breathing, first without retention and later with retention, to bring your entire system back into balance, the springboard from which you can then dive into meditation. Alternate nostril breathing, also known as *anuloma viloma*, is the process where you inhale through one nostril and exhale through the other in a systematic way to balance your nervous system. And how exactly does that work?

Remember the three main energy channels that run through your body: *ida*, *pingali*, and *sushuma*. The channel on the left, originating behind the left nostril and known as *ida nadi*, is associated with the feminine side in humans, the moon, and the Yin in you. When massaged with your breath, it ignites your parasympathetic system to relax your mental, biological, and physiological processes. This also activates the right side of your brain, thereby slowing down your mental processes and basically putting the reins on the mind.

The channel on the right side of your body, originating behind the right nostril and known for its abundance of heat, energy, and masculinity, is *pingala nadi* that is symbolized by the sun. It gives rise to energy, heat, strength, and creativity, all linked to the healthy characteristics of your sympathetic nervous system when it is not being chased by a shark. When your sympathetic nervous system is engaged in a healthy way and is in balance, it gives rise to unique creativity and positive energy. This channel stimulates the left side of your brain, the more extroverted side.

Therefore, when you engage in alternate nostril breathing, you literally alternate inhaling and exhaling through alternate nostrils to move closer to homeostasis. I won't explain the technique here as it is very easy to look it up on the Internet, but I will explain this: When you first start to use this technique, there should be no retention of breath and your inhale count should match your exhale count so as not to put stress on your nervous system by forcing *prana* through specific channels. However, once you have mastered this art of breathing, go ahead and retain, all you want in increments of two. But remember, never feel as if you are suffocating or in pain when you do so.

When practising *asanas*, you should always seek to keep your breathing constant. Please breathe through both nostrils, ensure that the inhale matches your exhale, and keep your focus on your breath to find comfort and stability in poses. Through the practise of *asanas*, you are preparing your body for meditation by ensuring all your systems are in balance. You don't want to be in a coma when you are in your asana practice, nor do you want to be so hyped up that you are merely partaking in an exercise.

Lastly, before I end today and go back to communicating with my community with the mycelium that lives under the shelter of Earth, I shall answer that question so often asked by humans: Why the nose and not the mouth? I am going to simplify this, as there is an entire science behind this and enough information to knock your brain out. The nose evolved to become an integral part of the respiratory system. When you inhale, the nose takes the air from the outside and warms it to your body temperature. It then hydrates it, so it goes down like a smooth martini, and then mixes it with nitric oxide. The latter not only kills off bacteria, but also increases the surface area of the alveoli, the little grape-like parts that hang off your lungs where the exchange of oxygen and carbon dioxide takes place. By increasing the surface area of the alveoli, your body can absorb

How Breath Works: The Trees Speak

more oxygen from the air you inhale and remove all the carbon dioxide when you exhale.

Remember how I told you that naturally each nostril opens and closes alternatively over a period throughout your day? That is because it is linked to your hypothalamus gland, which communicates with your nervous system to find balance. When the right nostril is open, it creates dominance in the sympathetic system. When the left nostril is open, it creates dominance in the parasympathetic system. So, in fact, your body naturally engages in alternate nostril breath all day every day. When you influence this system by practising *alunoma viloma pranayama*, you are, in fact, aiding a natural process.

Please note how the body does not breathe through one nostril for days, as humans often do with work and then on the weekend switch to the other one and go nuts. No, it does not because balance in everything is a daily process.

Nostril breathing also exercises your lungs and slows down your breath giving your lungs more time to facilitate the complete absorption of oxygen and eviction of carbon dioxide. The mouth is really for eating and drinking. It is also for those moments when you are being chased by a wild animal. I keep putting it like this: because originally your sympathetic system was really set up to fight for your life, to literally survive, or to hunt. it was not intended to be active in humans all the time.

When running, bench pressing something the size of a rhino, running around work and life like a chicken whose head just got cut off, you will breathe through your mouth. You will do this because you need your sympathetic system to kick in and do the following: metabolise sugar and carbs to release more energy into your muscles than usual; increase your heart rate, dilate your arteries, and so forth, so the rhino does not fall on your head and you do not pass out; and lastly remain alert from all the adrenaline being injected into you by your adrenal gland.

However, a large by product of sitting in your sympathetic system is faster, more shallow breathing. This, in turn, increases the level of carbon dioxide and lactic acid in the body. It is at this point that the mouth flips open to allow for more air to move in and out of your body, thus ensuring the quick release of built-up carbon dioxide and lactic acid in the blood. By doing this, your blood slowly moves back to its optimal PH, which was compromised by the high levels of lactic acid in it. Dramatic changes in the pH level of our blood are deeply harmful to your health. Your blood is the liquid that feeds your entire system.

It is the increase in carbon dioxide and not the decrease in oxygen that tells your respiratory system to drop your mouth open and move air in and out of you faster. Although breathing through your mouth makes exercise easier and requires much less lung strength, you should really try and keep it shut as much as possible.

Dumping loads of carbon dioxide also means that you are absorbing a lot less oxygen, which would be okay if you were a plant like us, but alas, you are not. Oxygen is your lifeline. We plants thank you deeply for all the carbon dioxide you keep offering us with your fast shallow breathing.

Lastly, mouth breathing keeps your body in its sympathetic system, and, by now, you know where that takes you. It is why when you practise Yoga, you should breathe through your nose. The nose is an undervalued genius."

With that Dragon Tree swayed her compact, stiff limbs and sighed, showering Corey in oxygen.

"Wow, so much knowledge you all have, so different from the intelligence we humans are constantly seeking. I feel as if knowledge are truths that we sacrifice for intelligence, which is the desire to know everything that is rooted in perspective. We humans put too much emphasis on intelligence over truth and knowledge. It is knowledge that will save our species and create a world that is more kind and connected. It is knowledge that should be taught in schools and to every child.

I am starting to understand that this work that you are teaching me, is something that should be given to children. It is only then that true and lasting change can come to my world and, by

How Breath Works: The Trees Speak

extension, the world beyond it. If we don't, we are doomed to keep conditioning children to grow up and repeat the same cycle that we adults are stuck on."

"Ahhh you are becoming wise, human." I laughed as I landed on Corey's shoulder. "Come, let us leave these happy beings and wander back toward your world."

"If I must. The stark contrast of this world to the one I live in has made me very aware just how much information and perspective is being pushed into my head constantly. Most have no basis in truth, and very little stems from original, contemplative, creative thought. As I have begun to filter what I place in my mind, I have begun to feel more free from fear." Corey swept his gaze and his smile across the cove and then bent his head in namaste.

"Thank you again for not trying to fix me and for providing me with awareness and the tools for me to heal and purify myself. I am, as always, grateful for the unconditional love you continue to give me every time we meet."

The cove bowed back at Corey, and I could feel their joy. Yoga was doing its magic, and we were deeply grateful. For it was in its magic that our survival rested.

18

Taming the Drunken Monkey Mind

As consciousness begins its journey toward its true self, it must do the following: First, it must open the human form, so it may begin to flow freely through the form. It does this through the medium of asanas. *Then it must learn to use* pranayama *to control the energy that feeds every cell in which consciousness resides. While doing this, it must begin to clean the mind by adhering to* yamas *and* niyamas. *These restraints and observances give rise to self-awareness through the purification of the mind. Each* yama *and* niyama *assists in the burning of illusions and the decolouring of impressions. Step by step, it peels back the attachments to all the* koshas. *Through meditation, it begins to hear itself, remove the* samskaras *and* karmas *that have burdened it, and finally be liberated to connect with the universal consciousness, the parent that birthed it and through which it shall connect to all its siblings, all living beings, as well as the infinite knowledge that sits within it.*

This is the story of meditation.......

I found Corey laying on the ground on his stomach and watching the tiny world pass him by. He allowed them to walk over him and rest on him. They were harmless, unless threatened, and so focused on their present path. He sat up as I landed on the ground beside him.

"They are beautiful, are they not?"

"They are," he replied, "and yet so many humans are scared of them. I am not sure it helps that we have labelled them as creepy crawlies and then developed a story around them that is not the kindest."

"Yes, it is an interesting human habit: creating all these narratives around nature that allow you to lazily believe that you have no impact or connection to any of us. In your movies and stories, we are often the villain. Our fires, storms, movements, and actions are all the source of terror and destruction to the

Taming the Drunken Monkey Mind

human. By portraying us in this way, you have succeeded in taking away our voice. You made us mute and then spoke for us with ignorance and lies. And why not? As long as you believe we are the destroyer and that you are not connected to us, you can keep eating us, chopping us down, polluting us, and caging us.

Many of us are on your weekly list. Yes Corey, even in your Amazon shopping. We arrive in pieces at your home, in boxes, as fibres, metals, etc. I hope you at least recycle us, so your children may grow up with greater odds of survival."

Corey lowered his eyes and said nothing. It was okay. He knew I was not judging, just raising awareness in him over and over again of our presence in his existence.

"Come, let's go sit with the trees. There is a breeze there, and you will find it easier to stay present in today's lesson. We are now starting to move into the last stretch of Yoga: meditation."

We slowly made our way to the family of trees and lay lazily among them. Everywhere we turned, there was nature reclined in a meditative state, only half aware of our presence for they had already begun to turn their senses inwards. Influenced by the energy around him, Corey's mind quieted, and his being shifted into his parasympathetic nervous system. It was under this blanket of blissful peace that I began the story of meditation.

"The next limb and first step toward meditation is *pratyahara*. It is the act of teaching your mind to withdraw from your senses and begin to focus on one thing and to learn to concentrate to establish peace with the mind. This cannot be done through running, swimming, or any physical act. It can only be accomplished by sitting and doing nothing. This is where Yoga begins to truly challenge you because the nature of the mind is to constantly move and be *rajasic*.

Ever notice when you sit in silence and observe your mind how many different and varying directions your mind goes? And how rarely the place your mind goes to is inside of you unless you are in pain or beating yourself up? Ever observe how you spend hours running around in your mind chasing a monkey who is high on speed? It mostly goes to places that are way beyond your control. It constantly shifts, and more often than not it is trying to figure out what someone else is thinking. As you well know, it is impossible to know what another person is thinking. I am not even sure the other knows what they are thinking or if they are just reacting. See how exhausting and pointless it all is to focus on that which is beyond our control?

The first stage of meditation is *pratyahara*. By definition, this is the process by which you begin to withdraw your senses from the objects that pull your senses toward them and then creates an attachment to them. For example, your sense of taste creates a desire to eat and then develops an attachment to the food, by adding the term 'I like' or 'I dislike' to it.

Therefore, in the practice of *pratyahara*, you are starting to teach the mind to concentrate, bring all the senses under control, and enter the journey of true introspection. Remember that the role of your senses is to provide proof that there is an outside world. If all your senses were switched off, you would be left with darkness, space, and silence with only your awareness to guide you. So, basically, you would be left connected to the Soul within you.

So, when a sense pulls you to something to satisfy itself, you respond by telling it 'no,' thereby gaining mastery over it. Seen this way, you begin to understand that your senses are what seek to constantly separate you from the Universal consciousness even though there is no difference between the individual and the Universe and you are, in fact, amid it.

True freedom, Corey, comes from mastering the mind and the senses. When you first start the practise of concentration, it is your senses that agitate and constantly prevent you from focusing on the infinite space in which we all exist. This is why

Taming the Drunken Monkey Mind

so many of you struggle with meditation: you have not first learnt to concentrate.

Now Corey, let me make this very clear. What most of you humans are doing at this stage is concentration not meditation. All those apps that you think you are using to engage in meditating are, in fact, trying to teach you to concentrate on one thing to quieten your mind. The transition to meditation occurs when your concentration on one object is so deep that you lose all awareness of time and space.

When you dream at night, you travel, experience things, feel things, and exit your bed as you enter a different realm of consciousness. Here, you experience things physically and mentally that are not really there at all. It is the same in your waking state: you perceive things that are not there because they are a construct of your mind. Only when you wake up from a dream do you know that it was a dream. Only when you are able to withdraw from your senses and wake up from the dream called life do you realise that life is merely an illusion created by your mind and that the truth lies beyond your mind. *Pratyahara*, therefore, is the first step toward your awakening from the illusion called life. Because everything is vibrating energy. Reality is merely how your mind perceives and structures that energy. Remember the story of the tire and how it is defined by who is looking at it.

Have you got a headache yet?" I squawked out loud in my eagle laughter. "I understand for many Humans this is a hard concept to grasp, and yet these days it is not only gurus, sufis, buddhists, and monks speaking this language, but also many neuroscientists, doctors, and physicists are beginning to participate in this same conversation.

There are many methods to *pratyahara*, but before you embark on them, there are some preconditions that must be met through the practice of *yamas*, *niyamas*, *asanas*, and *pranayama*. Your feelings and emotions should be *sattvic*. Your heart must be open as it is not only your mind, but also your heart that must engage in meditation, and your intention must be pure. When you first start this practise and you are so focused on your senses and their removal, your senses may become heightened, overactive, and very sensitive as they fight you to not be shut down. Remember the more attention you give something, the more power you offer it, the longer it will stick around. It is often at this stage that humans give up and descend back into the illusion called life.

In the wise words of that splendid human Buddha, let me share this with you:

Everything is transient, and yet, to the senses, everything seems to be permanent, which means that they cannot see reality. The same water does not flow in a river at any given spot. Everything is merely the motion of parts of something greater and made up of jumping and skipping particles. Every cell of the body constantly changes. Every atom of matter vibrates. Everything moves to something else. In this world the only constant is change on every level. But to the senses there is no change and life is never ending.

This is why humans struggle to accept death and believe it is something they can control and escape. They view death from their senses. If the soul is an angel of light, your senses are the devil.

Because where your senses really excel is in their want to satisfy desires. Humans live in the illusion that when a desire is met, fulfilment is satisfied. But all it does is fuel your desire for more fulfilment. The consequence of enjoyment is the generation of further desire to repeat the enjoyment. Always accompanying desire is suffering when a desire cannot be fulfilled or achieved or when the satisfaction of it leaves. Desire is like a fire, the more you feed it, the more it wants. This quote says it all: *Never is desire extinguished by the fulfilment of it.* It is your never-ending desire for pleasure that gives rise to your fear of death, as well as to possessiveness, jealousy, and that star player in your lives, suffering. You humans really need to put that player in the penalty box.

Taming the Drunken Monkey Mind

But something else much deeper than emotional insanity happens when you let your senses run amok. You create subtle psychic impressions in your subconscious mind. You create new *samskaras* and *karmas*.

When you first start this process of one pointed focus, the desires of your senses show themselves to be the greatest magicians of all. There are times when you will think, 'Aha I have tamed desire,' but really it is just lying low because maybe there is nothing to inspire it or it may be frustrated and exhausted and just taking a break. All the while, desire continues to scheme to create a circumstance in which it may rear its head again. When you are with us in nature, at a monastery, or at a temple, desires lose its strength and gives you the false impression that you have conquered it. Or it hides in depression, sadness, joy, or anger. Desires are sneaky buggers because in this state you blow the flames of desire to get you out of these low emotional states or to sustain a high.

Then there are moments when you once again think you have out-tricked desire only to find that the lack of desire for an external object has subtly replaced an attachment to it by engaging in fantasy and visualization to enjoy it in your mind. Or you have merely substituted desire for one thing with another. You humans are forever playing hide and seek with desire.

When you start this journey of training your mind, the journey is fraught with so much turmoil that your senses rebel. You feel lost and empty, and despair creeps in. When this happens, you find yourself asking 'what is the point of life? What is the point in engaging in a series of experiences that often leave you yearning for more?' These feelings will lead to unease in your body and manifest as lack of sleep, indiscriminate eating practices, and an overall feeling of lethargy. These occur as you seek to channel *prana* where it does not want to go, to control a mind that does not want to be controlled. But there are also moments of great joy that well up from within you when you least expect it. That reminds you why you are on this path.

Think of every training you have ever begun and how the start was always challenging. There was nearly always a moment when you just wanted to give up, but something in you pushed you forward. It is the same with *pratyahara*. Your mind wants you to give up, but if you listen carefully, your soul will propel you forward.

The best way to start concentration is with the external, and this may surprise you. We have spent months telling you to remove your focus on the external and move inward, but here the external has a benefit in that it provides a focus for your mind. Here are some examples of exercises for external focus:

Sit for a period of time and study Yoga, allowing your mind to concentrate on the study. Sit and listen to or read this book with full concentration. Basically, engage in one act at a time and be fully present in that one act rather than doing several acts at the same time or doing one act but thinking about another. For example, if you are washing a dish, be present in the whole act of washing it. Feel the water over your hands, feel the pot as you wash it, and basically be present in that very moment that is your life. There is joy to be found in every single act you do. You do not constantly need to be stimulated to feel great bliss in your life.

You can also begin concentration with meditation beads and chanting a mantra as you move from bead to bead giving your senses a focus. The candle meditation is very useful as well because it allows you to gently shift from the external to the internal. Light a candle in a darkened room and place it on a stand or blocks, so it is at the level of your heart. Keep your eyes wide open as you stare at the flame without blinking. When your eyes begin to water, close your eyes and focus on the image that appears between your eyebrows. Hold onto the image, and only when it disappears as you have lost concentration, open your eyes and start again.

From here, you can move on to focusing on the internal with visualisations. This is done by closing the eyes and focusing on a

Taming the Drunken Monkey Mind

chakra, the light between your eyebrows, or on an object placed in your heart, such as a lotus flower. When you have reached the point where you can concentrate on one thing comfortably over a long period of time, then you have reached the second stage of meditation: *dharana*. We shall get into *dharana* at our next meeting.

But before I end today, Corey, allow me to give you some homework on which to concentrate. Before you start every contemplation or meditation, enact these three principles. Enter into it with want for nothing. Acknowledge that you are nothing, that in this moment you are none of your roles or labels. And commit to doing nothing, to just be. As you enter into silence, your mind will seek to go anywhere and everywhere except into silence. That is okay. Instead of resisting, observe your thoughts with honesty and no judgement, knowing you are not your thoughts nor your emotions that for so long you have defined as your personality.

When witnessing your thoughts, ask yourself if the thought is useful or harmful to you. If it is harmful, take a moment to try and understand its origins. Observe the habits of your mind and the places it constantly seeks to go. These are mental habits you have created. Instead of sustaining the habit, let that thought stream go or transform it into a positive mental habit. For example, repeating a mantra such as 'I am love. I am enough just the way I am. I am light.'

The beginnings of this part of Yoga allow you to understand your mind and where it wants to constantly take you. Like any machine, you cannot fix it, transform it, or control it until you understand how it operates.

When a coloured thought rises, a like, a dislike, a lie, etc., try and bring it back to neutral by holding no attachment to it and then let it go. Ask yourself if the thought is a truth, fantasy, or gossip. Ask yourself if it is yours or was it given to you by another or media. It is only the colouring of your thought with *khelshas* that keeps you holding onto it. The only thoughts you should hang on to are truths.

When your mind pulls you somewhere, ask yourself if it is temporary or something you have attached to as permanent. For example, that you are ugly, fat, or a loser. Also ask yourself if you are mistaking a painful thought for pleasure, as you humans often do with love.

You will experience all of the above when you start to observe your mind, so do not panic; you are on the right path. The goal is not to suppress and bury what rises in the mind, but to still it by transforming thoughts back to their neutral state. In doing so, you will be burning the seeds from which they rose by not giving them attention or attaching yourself to them.

It is in this way that you begin to gently breaststroke your way around the Ocean, neutralizing negative thoughts, burning seeds, and allowing those thoughts that are useful to remain until the Ocean that is your mind and in which you swim around in all day is stilled. The small ego stops attaching itself to every thought and impression, the manas still, and the waves, the *vittris*, become flat. The *buddhi*, the intellect, stops trying to analyse everything and just listens.

And thus begins the process of breaking the cycle of karma that lives and breathes off your *samskaras*. You no longer live in the habit and behaviours that have been grooved into you by repeating them over and over again. Nor do you create new karmas. In every moment you enter, your behaviour will be guided by *yamas, niyamas,* and ultimately your consciousness. As you move forward in this journey, you will wake up one day and find that your mind always sits in one of these four states.

The first will be friendliness to all those that are joyful and are working to move themselves toward love and light. The second will be to have compassion for those who are suffering; they too have a story sitting in their conditioned mind. The third will be to always have reverence for those who have knowledge and are

Taming the Drunken Monkey Mind

taking the time to share it with you. And the last will be to have active indifference to all those who are evil and unkind in their actions.

I shall end today's lesson on a high. Corey, if you are really aware about what you put into your mind, one day all the seeds that sit at the bottom of your lake that give birth to thoughts will have been planted by you consciously and with awareness such that witnessing your mind will become a task you look forward to rather than fear. And in the stillness you will be able to move into the next step of meditation known as *dharana*.

"That was beautiful, Eagle," Corey exclaimed as he moved out of telepathy and back into his voice. "Thank you. I actually want to go home now to sit in silence and just observe my mind to know what is there. It is so much easier now that I understand that my mind is not me."

"You're most welcome, human Corey. Come let me fly you out of here, not literally. We would need dragons for that, and who knows? They may just show up one day."

Corey looked at me. He was unsure if I was speaking a truth or not, and then he smiled and let it go. He was beginning to understand that nothing was impossible. We turned to give gratitude and love to the cove, that was slowly awakening, and then slowly made our way back to the life of illusions.

"How are you doing?" I asked Corey. I was hoping he had learnt to answer that question with truth rather than the great human response: *I am okay.*

"Well, let's see. There are so many moments I feel joy and peace within me, but when I least expect it, that shifts quickly to doubt and fear. But those moments are becoming less as I am no longer feeding them my attention. But more than that, the fear of never seeing you again when this story is over keeps rearing its ugly head. I know we are near the end, and I so desperately want to ask you this: What will happen after the story of Yoga ends?"

I smiled at him, so proud that he had been able to articulate his emotions and thoughts.

"It gets easier, Corey. The mind never disappears, but your ability to control it and live above it grows. The more you surrender to the soul within, the less the external will pull you in all sorts of directions. As for us, I don't have the answer to that. I only know that at this moment, we are both exactly where we are meant to be. I have faith that this journey will continue for eternity, in many different forms, each as it is meant to be in that moment."

"I love your riddles, Eagle. You would do well to write a book on how to break free of a relationship, so it seems as if it is a gift to go separate ways. I know. I know. There is always a gift in all suffering."

"See? You no longer need me or the cove. The student has now become the master." I laughed out loud, happy at the light that was beginning to shine forth from him.

"That is not true. Eagle, I will always need you. Sorry, I meant want you. Wait. No, that is not right either because wants and needs are my senses and desires speaking. You know what I mean. Read my mind, will you?"

"I know what you mean. I feel the same way, but without the fear. We are deeply connected you and me. No amount of time, distance, or space will ever remove you or me from where our connection sits. In the other's heart."

19

Goodbye Illusion, Hello Universe

We had reached the last part of the meditation story, and the hopeful beginning of humans' journey into Yoga.

At the end of today's conversation, we would say goodbye to Corey. He was not ours to keep right now. A time would come for that, but for now he would have to return to his world and fulfill his purpose. He was only now starting to discover that his purpose was much bigger than capturing evil and more in-line with transforming evil.

He was beginning to understand that it was not the killing or jailing of evil or the quarantining of humans that would change this world. True lasting change is only possible with humans learning to live above their nature, to control desires, and to unattach from the material world. It is here that they would find joy and peace in their lives as every word, action, and behaviour that rose from them would arrive from a place of love and not fear. The connection to the soul within would allow for the connection to all living beings, even those outside of their species, to live a life where they never felt alone or unloved.

"Hello, Corey." I had chosen to meet him for our last conversation because I knew this would be hard for him.

"Hello, Beautiful. I knew you would come today. Is it really the last conversation we shall have?"

"I guess that depends on you. There are more ways for us to communicate than this." I landed on his shoulder to enjoy our last physical contact. I would miss his presence, but not in the way of suffering. "Also, now would probably be a good moment for you to engage in non-attachment."

Corey turned to look at me and smiled.

"You know, I have been contemplating a lot recently, and I have begun to wonder if maybe my purpose lies not in the law but in Jiu Jitsu. Did you know Ju Jitsu originated from Buddhist monks in India who used energy, rather than weapons of violence, to defend themselves? They, like yogis, understood the relationship between force and its influence over matter. Jiu Jitsu raises the *kundalini shakti*, the power that lives within each of us."

"Ah my human Corey, it is wonderful that you are beginning to move outside of your boxes and explore all that is open to you in this life. I am deeply pleased that by taking this journey you will discover your soul's purpose in this life. Now I want to say this to you before we enter the cove."

He stopped, and I perched on the rock in front of him. "Although this moment will transform into a new beginning for you, I will always be here for you when you need me. Just sit in silence and move into your meditation. It is here that you will hear me and feel me. I am a genius, really. I have opened a love in you for me so deep that you will have no choice but to meditate to see me again."

Corey burst out laughing and did not stop for minutes. His body shook, his energy danced, and for a moment I felt as if consciousness was showing itself. It was magnificent. "You actually are a genius, Eagle."

He then stopped and turned toward me. I could see the edges of his eyes glistening as tears began to escape from their jailer.

"Thank you, Eagle. Thank you for everything, for the light, the love, and for all the knowledge. If I do not move to a place of peace and bliss, then only I am to blame. You have given me all the tools, and now I am responsible for the path my life takes. If I continue to live a life devoid of pure love, then it will be because I chose fear and stopped loving myself. You have shown me what love is and for that I will forever be grateful to you. And when you die, if you could transform back into a human and show up in my life, well then, that will just be the magic I have been waiting for."

"Well Corey, you never know. We all live in a world where the impossible is possible. Now come, let us not sit in such sadness. It is a beautiful day, and all the cove has already entered into mediation waiting for this moment."

We had entered a silence that was beyond our greatest imagination. The whole cove lulled in a state of peace and love. It was tangible, and the air around us was set alight with thousands of beings all connecting to each other in this last meditation. We had decided to tell this last part of the story together, telepathically. For the entire story of Yoga lived in each of us.

"Come, Corey. Sit down at the base of Baobab and close your eyes. Begin by being aware of all the silence around you and your presence and connection to it. Gently drop out of your mind and into awareness. Take ten pause breaths: inhale, expand the belly, pause, expand the chest, pause, fill your head, and hold. Hold the air and energy in your head or solar plexus with relaxation, then exhale to your shoulders, pause, release the chest, pause, and then release the belly to finish the exhale. From there, engage in ten yogi breaths and then follow your natural breath and just listen. It is in this silence you will hear us."

I left him under the tree and flew onto the branch above him and closed my eyes.

"The last stage of meditation starts with your breath and ends with your pineal gland, located deep in the middle of your brain where the two halves meet. This master gland is shaped like a pinecone and is as small as a grain of rice. It is your light monitor. It sends information about light through your eyes to your hormonal centres. It has numerous important functions for the human form, but in Yoga it is most well known as the conduit to all the information that lays in the infinite space we call the Universe. It is your antenna.

In Yoga, it is known as your third eye and is located behind your *ajna chakra*, the *chakra* associated with light and illumination, your sixth sense. Its mantra is AUM. Through this antenna you are able to connect with the cosmic world without the filters of your past or your judgements. It is here that you engage in imagination and visualisation. When you tap into this gland, this *chakra*, you see the world with awareness and open eyes. You are open to the unknown, and you gain knowledge from beyond your senses. When this gland is calcified and shriveled and the *chakra* imbalanced, you feel blocked as if you are wading through a thick fog.

Only now is the Western world starting to appreciate what ancient traditions have known all along about the power of the pineal gland to connect.

- For Buddhists, the pineal is a symbol of spiritual awakening
- In Hinduism, the pineal is the seat of intuition and clairvoyance.
- For Taoists, the pineal is the *mind's eye* or *heavenly eye*.
- In ancient Egypt, there were numerous references to the third eye and the pineal region.
- And yes, even in the Bible, it is stated: *"The light of the body is the eye: if therefore thine eye be single, thy whole body shall be full of light."*

The pineal gland is called an eye because when you cut the gland in half the interior lining resembles the rods and cones found in the retina and has retinal tissue in it. How the ancients knew this without scanning machines is magical. In fact, the more technology humans have invented, the greater the distance you have created between your body, mind, and soul. Did you know, Human, that your form is actually a super computer with abilities way beyond today's technology that has been made redundant by technology? It's nuts, really.

To activate the pineal gland is no easy feat and doing so can harm you. Think of how often you have heard of some human having a bad trip from taking a drug that activated the pineal gland and led them to a place they did not want to go: into themselves. In the past, humans had healers, gurus, and shamans to guide you through this journey, but modern medicine and witch hunts have sought to eradicate and discredit them. This leaves you to navigate yourselves through a journey that is by no means simple and can create more harm than good if done without a teacher or healer.

The pineal gland is a nonendocrine transducer, which means it secretes a hormone when stimulated. The minute you open your eyes and allow light to enter, this gland starts to produce serotonin, a feel-good neurotransmitter. At the same time, it moves your brain waves from delta to theta to alpha to beta to cause you to once again realize you are in a physical body in space and time. When your brain is firing in beta brain waves, you put much of your attention on your outer environment, your body, and on time.

When night falls and it gets dark, an inverse process occurs. The inhibition of light sends a signal along the same route back to the pineal gland, which transmutes serotonin into melatonin. This slows down your brain waves from beta to alpha and makes you sleepy, tired, and less likely to want to think or analyse anything. As this happens, your attention shifts to your inner world rather than your outer world. Eventually, as your body falls asleep and goes into a catatonic state, your brain waves move from alpha to theta to delta to induce periods of dreaming as well as deep, restorative sleep.

As a transducer, the pineal gland can also send and receive energetic signals from wavelengths existing in the Universe, many of which resemble human brain waves, especially theta and delta brain. Therefore, when you meditate, what you are in fact doing is exerting mechanical pressure on the pineal gland, through breath, to create an electrical charge to turn the pineal gland into an antenna. This antenna in humans, however, works best when melatonin levels are at their highest: between 1am and 4am in the morning darkness. As a side note, did you know that the M in AUM is held the longest because its vibration serves to activate the pineal gland? Fascinating!

When the pineal gland is activated through breath, sound, and chanting, the brain has an orgasm, and melatonin transmutes into a chemical called benzodiazepine. This is the same drug group from which Valium (diazepam) is produced. In this state, your thinking brain, especially your emotional survival centre, the amygdala, is disabled to inhibit the influence of your emotions and thoughts.

From then onwards, if you can sit in this meditative state for a longer period, your frequency will begin to increase. As it does, more transmutations of melatonin will occur and start to bring your body into hibernation. As this happens, all your systems slow down and more energy is freed for the meditative process. The next step is the release of a powerful electric charge until, finally, you get to the chemical known as dimethyltriptamine (DMT), better known to you as Ayahusca.

It is here that you begin your communication with the quantum space where the unknown finally becomes the known. Now Corey, even if you never reach that stage, understand that every time you meditate, you create new neural pathways that not only open you up to new experiences and realities, but also move you further away from anxiety, depression, and any other popular labels for mental agitators.

Now that you understand the mechanics a little better, let us get back to the last stages of meditation. You will know when you have transitioned from *pratyahara* to the beginning of meditation, *dhyana*, because you have lost all sense of time and space, and even your own body. When the focus between you and the object you are focusing on remains continuous and unbroken by your senses and thoughts effortlessly, you will have moved into *dhyana*. In this stage, one hour will feel as if it were merely five minutes. As you move back into your waking state, you will have little sense of where you are. In your meditation, you will have lost all connection to your senses. There are some other signs such as feeling lightness in the body, visions of beauty or light, or hearing such sounds as the Ocean and bells. These are just some examples, but rest assured you will know when you have seen or heard it.

The last stage of meditation is *samadhi*, when you the observer becomes absorbed into that which you are observing. *Samadhi* is where all form dissipates and there is no separation, just oneness. Here, you the meditator will reach a full understanding of your true self and the universal consciousness. In doing so, you will have achieved full knowledge of the Universe and existence.

But even here, there are stages. We will only briefly summarize them as they too are large and would require a separate meditation to impart all the knowledge. Now, human, remember that the mind starts out my meditating on such gross objects as candles and then slowly on to subtler objects, like the vision of a lotus flower. When the mind can absorb itself into the object of meditation and understand and know its true energetic essence down to its simplest particle, then you will have entered *savitarka* meditation. Here, you will gain the inner workings and secrets of matter, and thereby gain mastery and power over them.

You know all those evil villains in superhero comics that have superpowers? Well, they are all meditators who have gained mastery over matter and energy but lack a moral foundation. This stage of meditation can be very harmful when achieved by someone who has not cleansed their mind.

The second stage is *savicara samadhi*, where you rise above time and space and can contemplate on the subtle without the aid of a gross object. For example, you can contemplate on love or the colour red and understand them fully as they are and not as defined by the conditioned mind. Here, you are able to give rise to thought while keeping the mind still. Here, you are aware that you are a form of energy meditating on a higher consciousness.

In the third stage, *sa-ananda samadhi*, there are no thoughts, no reflections, nor reasonings. The intellect is no longer present, and the mind is in a complete state of tranquility. All that is felt is joy and bliss.

Last is *sa-asmita samadhi,* the place where there is no I-ness. Here, the soul merges with *purusha*, the individual soul with the universal consciousness. In this stage, there are still *samskaras* sitting in the consciousness in seed form. In all four of these stages, the seeds of s*amskaras* are yet to be fully burnt. Hence, they are still susceptible to germination and give rise to disturbances and tendencies in the waking state.

Once you have reached the stage where the seeds remain, as they never really vanish, but are unable to germinate no matter how often you water them, you have attained *nirvikalpa samadhi,* where there is no more selflessness, no more "I want", just true liberation. Here, the human is completely unaffected by the form. These humans, known as *Jivanmuktas*, live and move among you humans. They look like you, but unlike you, they are completely *sattvic* in nature.

Human, you may not reach this final stage in this lifetime. It is a long and dedicated journey. But that is okay; you can still live a life of purpose and joy by achieving the lower states of meditation and engaging in *yamas, niyamas, asanas,* and *pranayama.* There is no need to denounce living in human societies. You can continue living your life, but now you will live it from a place of contentment, peace, and awareness. That alone makes the practice of Yoga worthy.

With that, we have come to the end of our journey together. There is nothing more left for us to say to you. We have given you the tools to create change; the choice is now yours. If you don't believe us, then all you have to do is try and see for yourself. You have nothing to lose and everything to gain. All we ask is that you start the journey and follow it to give it time to work its magic. We ask you to not give up so easily and to choose you, to choose us, to choose a life of love, kindness, compassion, and sharing over one of fear, anxiety, suffering, and chaos.

Because our fate, the fate of your species as well as our own fate, rests in you.

20

The Awakening

Corey opened his eyes and for longer than a moment had no concept of where he was or how long he had been sitting in meditation under the tree. He took a deep inhale and exhale, and then he looked around, remembering where he was.

He was sitting under a baobab tree at the edge of a cliff overlooking the Ocean. He was surrounded by trees, plants, the Earth, and so much silence. As he became aware of his body and his surroundings, he remembered following an Eagle who had flown around him for minutes before leading him to his place. For some reason unbeknown to him, he had been overcome by a deep need to meditate, so he had sat at the base of this tree that had summoned him.

He looked into his bag and found his watch; he had been sitting here for over an hour, and yet it had seemed he had been away for much longer than that. He smiled as he realised that he had reached a new level of *samadhi*, one in which the Universe had spoken to him in many different forms and provided him with knowledge and truth. It was true, all that he had heard and read about. In connecting to his true self, he had connected to all the infinite knowledge in the Universe and discovered the truth about Yoga.

It had all seemed so real, more real than his present reality of being awake. He closed his eyes. He wanted to go back to that place where he had experienced a love like none other, a place that had left him feeling joyous. As he tightened his eyes and asked them to bring forth the cove, he heard the Eagle. For a moment, he thought, "wow, that was easy." But as the squawk continued, he opened his eyes and looked into the blue sky above.

It was the same Eagle, the one he instinctively knew had led him to his place that he was struggling to leave. Unsure of what lay

The Awakening

in the next moment, he watched her as she gently swooped down from the sky and landed on the tree above. For a moment, they both stared at each other. Corey half expected her to say, "Hello Corey," in that great Indian accent of hers.

Then she spread her wings and lifted off the tree to fly circles around him. He knew she was asking him to follow her, so he did. She had, after all, led him here. He slowly untangled his body, so grateful for *asanas*, and began to follow the eagle. As he made his way across the cliff and down to a little beach, he stopped in his tracks. There, on the beach below him, sat a vision of beauty. A brown-skinned woman was sitting on a Yoga mat surrounded by a spectrum of humans.

Mesmerised, he sat down on a rock and listened to what she was saying. He watched the Eagle swoop over her head. As it did, she raised her head and smiled at the Eagle as if they were one, and then she spoke:

"Hello, Eagle, so nice to see you again. Thank you for coming to visit and reminding these humans that you are connected to them." She bowed to the Eagle as it glided back out into the Ocean.

He could see the look of amusement on her students. They obviously had spent time with her. None of them looked at her as if she were crazy. He listened as she began to speak to them, and what he heard left his heart with a yearning to love her. She spoke with an Indian accent, the same one Eagle had spoken to him in his meditations. How was it possible? And then he smiled, remembering Eagle's famous words that in Yoga the impossible was always possible.

Her words mesmerised him. It was as if the contents of his meditations were spilling out into his waking world. Here is what he heard flow out of her being:

"My greatest wish for all of you is that at the end of our time together this week, you will have a greater understanding of what Yoga is. You will understand that it is not an exercise or a cult, but a way of life that when coupled with a healthy diet will literally change your life forever. If change is what you seek, of course. Because as you have seen, it is all connected. What we feed our body, our mind, our senses all have a deep and profound impact on how our lives play out.

Our human form is a manifestation of nature and therefore transient. Only your soul is immortal and part of the larger consciousness, known as the Universe. In the coming week, I hope to give you both the awareness and the tools to be healthy and to connect you to more realities than the one you live in now. You define your reality by what you project out onto it. It is not the external world that defines who you are and how your life will play out, but your response to that world. Changing the external will not incite internal change, but changing yourself will change the external to reflect who you are becoming.

So yes, Sonia and Paola, changing your clothes, your hair, your partner or your car will not really create lasting change in your life."

He watched them laugh with her as if they had all known each other for a lifetime. Even he felt a connection to her, although he had never met her. Or had he? He pulled his attention back into the moment. He wanted to hear more of her thoughts.

"Now, should you choose to not follow the path of Yoga or any path that espouses internal change, you will forever be limited in the life you lead. Additionally, you may never attain your highest potential or know your true purpose.. This is not a threat, merely a truth.

I know many of you listening to me feel helpless and powerless to create change in the world. Well, it may surprise you to know that the Universe, actually hangs out in your form and is just sitting around waiting for you to take the journey to it, so it may reveal the unimaginable power that lives within you.

You know, my friends, we say be kind to strangers, even those who are not kind to you, because you are connected to every

The Awakening

living being. And if for a moment in time, you can cause even the slightest shift in someone through an act of kindness and compassion, you will change the path of that person, even if just by a degree. That slight change will change the trajectory of life on this planet, which will then resonate out into the rest of the Universe. Because remember: everything that happens in your life is a result of or influenced by the actions of every other living thing on this planet and vice versa.

This has been by far the greatest gift Yoga has given me. It has disabled my ego and pride, and in its place opened a fountain of love that flows over all that cross my path. In response to all I give out, I have been shown so much love from strangers, friends, animals, and the Universe. There is not a day that passes that I don't have a moment of being stunned by how much love there is out there when it is given a safe space and the confidence to reveal itself. I am shown how we are all so deeply connected to each other under all our superficial differences.

Yoga has taught me that when people begin to drain my energy to a point where it is not healthy for me, I can remove myself from those relationships to be kind to me. Because Yoga is also about being kind to yourself and loving yourself from a place of light not ego. And sometimes being kind and loving to yourself, means having to say 'no' as well as learning to accept 'no.'

I hope through the story of Yoga, which I shall begin to teach you from your mat, you may understand that there is no shortcut or app to change. To connect to every living thing, to have a multitude of beautiful lives in this lifetime, will take work. There is not a day that goes by where I don't have to do the work by either coming to my mat, meditating, self-observing or adhering to *yamas* and *niyamas*. Don't get me wrong; there are days when I fall off my mat, and I just want to give up and descend back into hole from which I climbed out off. But then something happens: a perfect stranger shows me an unexpected love and kindness, an animal seeks my company, or a river of gratitude and happiness washes over my heart to remind me why I am on this journey.

This path is so hard because our conditioned mind is strong, especially if you get on this path when you are older. If everyone understood Yoga and started practising from a young age, we could bring our world back into balance within a generation. It would not matter how many humans there were in the world, because each and every one of us would live in balance and harmony with our planet. We would lead from our souls and not from our senses and desires.

We would stop interfering with the process of life. We would accept our journeys and live lives devoid of chronic, harmful stress. And as a result, we would most likely die healthy deaths. But most importantly, we would live life, accept death, and live in a world of unbound imaginative creativity.

So many of us fail to ever access the unique creativity that sits within. We are a manifestation of the Universe, and within each one of us there exists the creativity and power that led to creation. Look at the natural world and its creative magnificence. How often have you looked at something like the Victoria Falls and been speechless? We have that same creativity within us to create beauty that lives in coherence with its environment. Just think what our world could look like if we were all able to access that unique creative energy and use it for the betterment of our existence rather than for financial gain. We would live in forests and gardens, and there would be no waste, no pollution, nor cars. Best of all, we would live in a world of love and contentment, where thy neighbor may just be a hippo.

It takes great strength to move against the stream and not let others' fears, judgements, and perspectives beat you back into the box. It takes courage to literally dare to be different, so the next time you hit a wall in your life, don't just lay down and give up or keep hitting it. Instead stop, step back, and understand where that wall came from because most likely it is a wall you have built that comes from your past, your own karma.

The Awakening

Yoga has taught me all this as well as shown me how to observe and control my mind and behaviours. To harness the potential of my energetic body to connect to all the different frequencies out there and to truly know that what I give out in my intentions, my energy, will be reflected back to me in my reality.

Yoga has taught me to understand the power of mantras when repeated. Each word containing a vibration and energy that shifts my vibration and unblocks me. To understand that such rituals as fasting are about learning to reign in my senses and control my desires. Yoga has taught me about the power of thought not only when sent out into the world, but also when creating a new garden of thoughts and ideas in the mind.

Too often we are taught rituals and told to engage in behaviours without understanding why we do them. We follow them blindly, and as a result end up not entertaining change. This is why so many wars are still fought in the name of religion, why so much division and hatred between humans remains: you are blind followers rather than enlightened leaders in your own life.

Only acts done with full knowledge translate into deep change, and only in change can we all influence our destiny set out by our *karmas*. It is just too easy to blame the world and others for your lives because to accept responsibility for your life is to acknowledge all your fallibilities, your insecurities, and your fears. When you do this, you then understand that every bad thing that ever happened to you happened for a reason. It was not random. Instead of allowing those acts to drown you, Yoga asks you to learn from them and use them to change. Yoga asks you to say thank you to all those that hurt you because they came to teach.

There can be no change without vulnerability, because only when we are vulnerable are we open to change. Otherwise we are locked behind walls, where we speak change but don´t allow for it. There can be no change without acceptance or surrender. Lastly, there can be no change without accepting who you are in this moment, with the understanding that it does not mean that is who you will always be. You can be anyone you want to be."

With that, she placed her hands together and asked her students to do the same. They finished with the AUMs that were still resonating in his head.

It was then that he knew that he had found the love he had experienced in his meditations. Eagle really was a genius for she had led him to a soul filled with light and love. In his heart, he knew that to love someone like her, he would have to engage in a love devoid of fear. He would have to practise Yoga.

He slowly stood up and walked down the beach. He was waiting for the students to wander off before he approached her.

"Hi, I am Corey. I have sat listening to you and was wondering if I could walk with you for a little while. I have just come out of the most magnificent meditation, and when I did, your Eagle led me to you."

She burst out into a laughter that made his heart light up. "Yes. The Eagle, I love her. She came to me when I most needed to hear nature and then continued to appear every time I needed to be reminded that I was free and only my mind enslaves me."

She paused, stared into his eyes for a moment, and then smiled. "Sure. Let's walk, so I may discover why my friend the Eagle has brought you to me, if you have a message for me, or if you are the one I have been asking the Universe for in my meditations. Come, you can walk me back to my Yoga studio."

He fell into step with her as she began to walk down the beach. For several moments they walked with silence between them. He knew she was taking a moment to let her energy meet his, and then she turned to him and said, "By the way, my name is Sheena."

In that moment, Corey knew the magic of Yoga had begun. As his eyes traveled across Sky, along Ocean, down at Earth, and then gazed at the trees in the distance, he gently bowed his head

The Awakening

as he felt the impossible meeting the possible and whispered, "thank you".

How the Impossible Became Possible
The True Story of an Indian Girl From Criminals to Yogi

Desert Island in the Middle of the Atlantic Ocean, 2021

Corey replicated Houdini's greatest act and disappeared as quickly as he had appeared in my life. He had arrived to apprehend a fugitive during the Covid pandemic, when there were no planes coming in or out of the island.

We had spoken for a total of thirty minutes over three separate encounters, and then poof! He had returned to this homeland. Days later he messaged me.

"Hi. Sorry I could not come to a Yoga class, but I had to return home. But I would love to get to know you a little better."

I, of course, considered him insane. He had been here for nearly six weeks, and he had never sought to know me in all that time. However, I was intrigued, and thus conceded, not fully knowing what a journey I was about to embark on. A world that I could never have imagined. It contained all the boxes I would never have opened and entered by my own volition. The box of religion, warrior, cop, guns, trauma, conservative, private, and, well, the list was long.

What ensued from that one askance to know me more was a journey that would ignite my world and fueled a journey into the depths of Yoga. There was no other way I could be with him but as a yogi. It was the most challenging path I could have chosen to walk with another, but I did because he was who I had been waiting for. The one that sat on the flip side of the coin to the other one.

The other one. A grown boy who I had met when I was 14 and living in Zambia. He had been chosen by my soul to fulfill a *karma* that had been created before I was born. Such was our connection, that our journey would span three decades, four continents, rape, death, and the most ambitious form of love I could then imagine. That was until I met the agent. These two men would change my life forever, and the lives of every single human that walked into my Yoga studio from the day I choose to give everything up, except for Yoga.

The Beep in the Jungle, 2003

I had woken up before the sun and walked across the camp to find a signal on my phone. I am not sure why? Those few who had my number had been told not to contact me, no matter what. I was in the middle of the African bush, and no matter what you wanted to tell me, there was nothing I could do about it. So why burden me with something that was beyond my control?

I had not switched on my phone since I had chosen to spend eight months in the bush, away from Indians and a western material culture that had begun to suffocate me, since the death of my father. As I stood there in the open plains, surrounded by a herd of buffalo, I was mesmerised by the African sun, a ball of orange flames simmering in its own aura, rising from the horizon.

I knew exactly why I was standing there at 5.30am in the morning, with my hand in the air trying to find the smallest of signals; it was because of the dream. The same one I'd had five years ago, followed by the reappearance of Dexter.

Dexter is every Indian mother's worst nightmare. Mixed race, drug dealer, stolen car launderer, and criminal extraordinaire who was part of the largest illegal organisation in Southern Africa. A man who would taint my chances of ever meeting a good Indian doctor or engineer in our small Indian community. A man who would blacklist me from entering Indian households and befriending other Indian girls my age.

Then it beeped and shattered the stillness that surrounded me. It beeped again, and, as if on cue, the sun seemed to suck all the energy from the dry, cracked earth. Everything went silent. For what seemed like hours but could have only been seconds, there was just the beep echoing off the thorn trees that surrounded the camp. Every animal in a five-mile radius seemed to be holding its breath, waiting for me to breathe.

With my mouth flipped open, searching for extra oxygen, and the feeling of an oncoming heart attack in my chest, I opened the texts.

Hi.

Followed by:

You there?

He had found me again. The sounds of the bush brought me back to the present, and I thought, "not this time."

It had taken me nearly a year to recover from the last dream and what had followed, so I switched off the phone and wandered down to the watering hole to find better company than my ghosts. The small watering hole that lay opposite our kitchen and open lounging area was often frequented by giraffes, warthogs, and the occasional antelope. As I wandered down the ad hoc path created by hiking boots, I wondered if he was in a game reserve as well. For as long as I had known Dexter, he had loved the bush and Indian girls.

I understood the draw of the wild for him. I had started going into the bush when I was fourteen and had kept returning since then. It was one of the many gifts my unique Indian father had given me. Love for the wilderness, which for an Indian girl was rare. In fact, everything about my life as an Indian was different. A story that began with my ancestors, whom in their own little way had all moved against the stream.

On approaching the small watering hole, I was not disappointed. Standing elegantly upright were two giraffes feeding off the acacia trees that acted as both food and umbrella. As I watched them, my mind drifted back to Dexter.

He came from a world that had been as foreign to me as the Milky Way. But not foreign to the Indian boys who lived in Zambia. It never ceased to impress me how in one household, one culture, one religion, men and women lived two completely separate realities, where one was a prisoner and the other the warden. It was why Dexter's world appealed to me. In it, I discovered freedom as I had never experienced before. Once I had tasted it, I knew I would cheat, lie, steal, and use others to keep returning to it.

Fearing the uncontrollable obsession that Dexter bought out in me, I yanked my mind back into the present and focused on Baixinhas (B), our local Rhino. If she could survive years of stress and loneliness on a celebrity ranch, I could get past this. Not wanting to keep B waiting for her bath, I slipped the phone into my pocket and headed over to the scary kitchen. It was equipped with basic kitchen utensils and a thatched roof, from which two black mambas had dropped onto our eating table a few weeks ago.

Printed in Great Britain
by Amazon